SPORTS NUTRITION

The Ultimate Nutrition Bible for Enhancing Athletic Performance, Supporting Quick Recovery, and Becoming a Faster, Better, and Stronger Athlete

MATT JORDAN

©Copyright 2017 by Matt Jordan- All rights reserved.

This document is presented with the desire to provide reliable, quality information about the topic in question and the facts discussed within. This Book is sold under the assumption that neither the author nor the publisher should be asked to provide the services discussed within. If any discussion, professional or legal, is otherwise required a proper professional should be consulted.

This Declaration was held acceptable and equally approved by the Committee of Publishers and Associations as well as the American Bar Association.

The reproduction, duplication or transmission of any of the included information is considered illegal whether done in print or electronically. Creating a recorded copy or a secondary copy of this work is also prohibited unless the action of doing so is first cleared through the Publisher and condoned in writing. All rights reserved.

Any information contained in the following pages is considered accurate and truthful and that any liability through inattention or by any use or misuse of the topics discussed within falls solely on the reader. There are no cases in which the Publisher of this work can be held responsible or be asked to provide reparations for any loss of monetary gain or other damages which may be caused by following the presented information in any way shape or form.

The following information is presented purely for informative purposes and is therefore considered universal. The information presented within is done so without a contract or any other type of assurance as to its quality or validity.

Table of Contents

INTRODUCTION 1

PART I: THE BASICS OF SPORTS NUTRITION 2

    ENERGY REQUIREMENTS 3

    ENERGY NUTRIENTS 7

    SUPERFOODS FOR ATHLETES AND PERFORMANCE 19

    VITAMINS AND MINERALS 25

    SUPPLEMENTS FOR ENHANCING ENDURANCE PERFORMANCE 30

    FLUIDS AND ELECTROLYTES 33

    ENERGY TO FUEL 36

PART II: THE ULTIMATE MEAL PLAN FOR ENDURANCE ATHLETES 41

    PLANNING WISELY 42

    THE 4-WEEK MEAL PLAN 45

PART III: RECIPES FOR ATHLETIC PERFORMANCE 74

    BREAKFAST 74

    LUNCH 84

    DINNER 100

    SNACKS 115

CONCLUSION 124

PREVIEW OF TRIATHLON TRAINING BY MATT JORDAN 125

    WHY SO DISCOURAGED? 125

Introduction

Whether an occasional runner, an aspiring swimmer, or an Olympic triathlete, one thing is certain, in order for you to get to the finish line and achieve your athletic goal, you will need a proper source of energy to fuel and power your exercises.

Playing a huge part in the performance of every athlete, properly balanced nutrition is just as essential as an adequate amount of exercise is. And yet, many athletes tend to overlook the benefits that eating a balanced meal can bring to their endurance and performance and choose to overindulge in not-so-healthy choices instead. This mostly happens because people are under the illusion that a healthy diet is a boring and tasteless diet by default. Well, quite the opposite is true, actually.

If you are an athlete that wishes to reach his/her peak performance, then you have definitely come to the right place. Being the ultimate nutrition guide that every athlete can benefit from, this extremely helpful book will guide you through your active journey of becoming a better, faster, and stronger athlete.

Offering you an in-depth explanation of what sports nutrition is and why it is important, revealing the ultimate tips and tricks for staying energized during and post workouts, and providing you with a carefully created four-week meal plan for every athlete, as well as some yummy recipes to stack your recipe folder with, this book will be your shield against injuries and the best power and endurance charger.

Are you ready to see how far you can actually go?

Part I: The Basics of Sports Nutrition

Sports nutrition is anything but complicated. Just because you, as an endurance athlete, will need more energy to get you going throughout the day than the average person, doesn't mean that your diet should be overwhelming.

Besides the need for an increased amount of fuel, the athlete's diet is not really that different than the normal healthy diet that most nutritionists recommend. If you think that embarking on a super active and physically demanding journey means that you should count every single calorie and not enjoy the taste of your meals, you cannot be more wrong.

After mastering the non-overwhelming guidelines for the right sports nutrition that can be found in this chapter's section, you can freely enjoy eating without worrying yourself whether or not your muscles are receiving adequate energy.

ENERGY REQUIREMENTS

Ensuring that they have the needed energy to endure the toughness of the physical activity is every athlete's priority. Even the tiniest deficit between the energy consumed and the energy output can not only lead to poor performance, but it can also be the cause of many unwanted complications and injuries.

It has been scientifically proven that athletic performance is based on nutritional intake, and as such, it varies for different people. Those who eat less than recommended are far from reaching their athletic goals, but so are those that eat more than they should. When it comes to meeting the energy requirements for boosting your performance, balance is the key.

Those athletes that are able to reach and then continue maintaining their peak performance are those that know how to best provide the requisite energy needed to fuel their physical activities. These are the ones that can convert the energy stored within their bodies into the fuel needed to endure and execute tough and physically demanding workouts. But besides what is obviously crucial for them to be able to achieve their goals, and that is the consumption of the right type of calories, the correct amounts of the calories consumed also play an important part in the quality of their athletic performance.

As humans, we need energy to be physically active just like a car needs fuel to get from point A to point B. We consume that energy in the form of calories that we ingest from different foods, and then we use that amount of energy to fuel the necessary functions such as breathing, moving, etc. Obviously, the more calories and energy we lose during physical activity, the higher our body's demand is for this type of energy. That being said, it is pretty obvious that super active athletes have a higher calorie demand than the average person.

To explain this in the best way possible, I will use a simple math formula:

Calories consumed—calories needed = net calories

When we eat more calories than required, our net calories are positive, which means that there are extra calories stored that later get used as fat, therefore, we gain weight. When we eat fewer calories than required, our net calories are negative, which means that the stored energy levels are lowered, therefore, we lose weight. Neither positive nor negative net calories will result in achievement of our athletic goals. In order for an athlete to perform optimally, his or her net calories should be in a neutral state, or zero, meaning that the calories consumed should roughly match calories needed.

But the question remains what is our ideal calorie intake? How do we know what our ideal net calorie amount is? Unfortunately, since we are all different, we cannot exactly say that there is a one-of-a-kind formula by which every athlete should plan their meals.

The factors that determine the athlete's requirement for energy are based on many factors, such as the type, intensity, and frequency of the training, the body composition, the goals, etc. As I said, there isn't really a one-of-a-kind recommendation that will show whether or not your calories are balanced. There are different formulas that can be used for this purpose, but none of them are set in stone. You should try many different tools to check if you are achieving the right balance of energy with your weight, appetite, fat percentage, and your overall health in general.

Basal Metabolic Rate (BMR)

Our bodies use approximately 60 percent of the calories consumed in order to be able to properly function and finish all of the necessary processes when we rest. The number of calories we burn while we rest is called our BMR or Basal Metabolic Rate. People that have a leaner body mass have a higher BMR, which means that they burn calories faster. That is why overweight people are encouraged to eat more smaller meals during the day because, that way, the body can burn more calories since 30 percent of the energy is used for physical activity and 10 percent is used during digestion.

You can determine your BMR with this formula:

Men
BMR = 66.47 + (13.75 x Weight(kg)) + (5.0 x Height(cm)) — (6.75 x Years of Age)

Women
BMR = 665.09 + (9.56 x Weight(kg)) + (1.84 x Height(cm) — (4.67 x Years of Age)

If this seems like too much of a hassle, you can simplify this formula with this simple rule:

If you are male, you can calculate your BMR by multiplying your weight (in pounds) by 11. If you are female, multiply your weight by 10. That means that men should eat 11 calories for each pound they weigh and women 10.

For instance, if you are a man and you weigh 200 pounds, your ideal daily intake should be 2,200 calories.

Sterling - Pasmore Equation

This is a simple equation for determining BMR based on the composition of your body.

$$BMR = Lean\ Body\ Mass\ (pounds) \times 13.8\ calories$$

That means that your body needs 13.8 calories consumed in order to be able to support a pound of your lean body mass.

If you don't know your lean body mass you can calculate it based on your other measurements:

$$Body\ Fat\ Percentage \times Scale\ Weight = Fat\ Mass$$

$$Scale\ Weight - Fat\ Mass = Lean\ Body\ Mass$$

Daily Energy Requirements for Athletes:

Athletes need balanced nutritional intake in order to fuel their athletic performance. However, the requirements are not the same for all athlete types.

- Sedentary men and women that are not pregnant should consume about 31 calories for every kg of their body weight.

- Men and non-pregnant women that are recreational athletes should consume about 33 to 38 calories per every kg of their weight.

- Endurance athletes should consume from 30 to 50 calories per each of the kg of their weight, depending on the type and intensity of their training.

- Strength-trained athletes should consume from 30 to 60 calories per each kg of their weight, depending on their training.

ENERGY NUTRIENTS

The capacity of athletes to perform demanding physical activities is mainly determined by their ability to rally the levels of stored energy and then shove them to power the contractions of the muscles. In order to perform these activities efficiently, the athlete needs to have stored energy available. If there is a lack of stored energy, the athlete will not be able to fuel the body and the muscle contractions, which will not only lead to poor performance but also fatigue and probably some more serious injuries.

The major sources of energy and fuel for the muscles are the three macronutrients: carbohydrates, fats, and protein.

Carbohydrates for Energy Production

There is no doubt that carbohydrates are the real superstar when it comes to fueling the body with the right amount of energy needed for it to function properly. Carbohydrates or carbs serve the most of the important roles in the body, and it is the source of 60 % of the total energy in the daily diet of an endurance athlete such as runners or triathletes.

Not only athletes but people of all ages and exercise abilities will benefit from implementing carb-rich foods into their diet. However, the giant confusion that has been floating around lately encourages people to go against the grains and bans this macronutrient from their plates. If you too are confused about the role that carbs play in your diet and the benefits that it may bring, then this chapter will eliminate all confusions and make you understand why and which carbs should be an inevitable part of your journey to reaching your athletic goal.

Types of Carbohydrates

Dumping all carbohydrates into the same group is a mistake since not all carbs are created equal. In order to understand just how important their presence in your diet is, you must first learn about the different types of carbohydrates.

As the name itself suggests, carbohydrates contain carbon and water with the formula of CH_2O. They can be classified into different groups based on a couple of factors:

- The type of carbohydrates in the food;
- The type of commercial processing that it has been through;
- The glycemic or blood sugar response to the carb within the body;

The simplest way of classifying carbohydrates is into simple and complex carbs. The other classification is into monosaccharide, disaccharides, oligosaccharides, and polysaccharides. However, for the sake of convenience, I will simplify the process and combine these two classifications.

Simple Carbohydrates are monosaccharide and disaccharides. The monosaccharide represent the simplest form of sugars such as glucose, fructose, and galactose. These sugars are single- sugar molecules. The disaccharides are double- sugar molecules and the common sources are table sugar or sucrose, milk sugar or lactose, honey, and corn syrup.

This type of carbohydrates is called simple because they are easily broken down into sugars during digestion in order to be immediately used as energy. For instance, table sugar, honey, and corn syrup contain both fructose and glucose, however, not in equal amounts. During digestion, table sugar breaks down into 50 % of both glucose and fructose. Honey breaks down into 31 % of glucose, 38 % of fructose, 10 % of other forms of sugars, 10 % of water, and 4 percent of other particles. Corn syrup converts into 55 percent of fructose and 45 % of glucose. The line is that both monosaccharide and disaccharides are eventually converted into glucose which is transferred through our bloodstream in order to fuel the brain, as well as the muscles.

Fruits and veggies also contain sugars but in many different forms and proportions. Because of the fact that absorbing different types of sugars at different rates and proportions lead to better energy absorption during physical activity, it is recommended that when buying sports drinks you pay close attention to what the label says and buy only those that contain multiple types of sugar.

Also, when buying drinks, make sure that you avoid fructose when possible (mostly soda and other soft drinks) since research suggest that fructose is absorbed differently than glucose, in a way that contributes to producing more fat and favors weight gain.

And while honey is considered to be healthier than white sugar, keep in mind that it is in no way superior when it comes to nutrients, vitamins, or health benefits. Any form of sugar, whether it is refined sugar, corn syrup, honey, maple syrup, brown sugar, etc. it provides none nutritional value whatsoever. If you are looking for a way to load up on energy, you can do it with much healthier ingredients, since all carbohydrates get eventually broken down into glucose.

Complex Carbohydrates, as you have probably already guessed, are oligosaccharides and polysaccharides. This type of carbs is formed when there are three or more simple carbs linked together in a long, complex chain. Just like the simple carbs, complex carbohydrates get also broken down into sugars but in a different way. During digestion, complex carbs are broken down into glucose slower than simple carbs, which leads to a longer lasting energy. Besides, complex carbohydrates are not 'empty' carbs such as the simple ones; besides the energy that they provide, they are far healthier since they are loaded with essential nutrients such as vitamins, minerals, and fiber. The complex carbs are mostly made of starches. And in case you have no idea what 'starch' is, it is a polysaccharide that plants store as extra energy. An interesting fact is that veggies become starchier as they ripen, while fruits tend to convert the starch into sugars as they get older. Just an important fact to have in mind when going grocery shopping.

Complex carbohydrates can bring a number of benefits that will positively affect not only your athletic performance, but overall health as well. Some most common sources of complex carbs are barley, bulgur, lentils, oatmeal, potato, split peas, green peas, wheat, starchy vegetables, quinoa, whole grains, beans, brown rice, wild rice, etc.

Remember that although fruits and vegetables are simple carbs, they are super nutritious and contain fiber, minerals, and vitamins, which make them more complex in nature and should be consumed on a daily basis.

The Glycemic Index and Glycemic Load

As I said, all carbs get eventually broken down into glucose, making glucose the final product of the carb digestion. What does that mean? That means that the levels of glucose in the blood increase after the carb-loaded food is digested. However, just like not all carbs are equal, the same way all carbs do not affect the blood glucose levels equally. Some of the carbs get broken down into glucose quickly and result in a blood sugar spike, while some of them, even though contain a high carb intake, may not cause any significant elevation of the blood glucose. How the carbohydrates consumed will affect the blood sugar depends on their Glycemic Index. The rule is that those carbs that have a higher Glycemic Index are quickly absorbed causing a rapid blood sugar rise, while those carbs with a low Glycemic Index are slowly absorbed and cause only a small increase in the blood sugar levels.

The Glycemic Index is mainly based on how 50 g of carbs in a food will affect your blood glucose levels. And while the Glycemic Index was originally developed to help people with diabetes manage their blood sugar, this complex system is not the best indicator of how the food will affect the blood sugar. You see, the Glycemic Index shows us how rapidly the carbs are absorbed and broken down into sugars, but it doesn't take into account how many carbs there are in the food consumed. For that, we use a different ranking system called the Glycemic Load.

For instance, a 60-gram piece of banana cake with sugar has a Glycemic Index of 47 and a Glycemic Load of 14. On the other hand, a 60-gram piece of banana cake made without sugar has a Glycemic Index of 55, but a Glycemic Load of 12. You see, even though the banana cake without sugar has a higher Glycemic Index, it will not raise the blood sugar levels as much as a piece of banana cake with sugar will.

Now, whether or not you should obsess about the Glycemic Load or Glycemic Index of the food, is a different thing. Some athletes believe that eating low GL foods will provide them with sustained energy for the long exercises. Some also believe that eating high GL foods immediately after a workout is a great way to recover as it will refuel the muscles which will lead to better performance over the next days.

If you ask me, I say do not get too carried away with the Glycemic numbers, but try to enjoy the food you eat. There are a lot of factors that can affect the Glycemic Load such as the fact that we all have a different response to different foods, the place where the food was grown, whether the food has added fat or not, the way that it is prepared, etc. The best way in which you will find which foods bring you the energy of highest quality is through a process of trial and error. And while the high Glycemic Load foods are the best energy sources for those athletes that train hard, try not to get too obsessed. See how your body reacts after eating certain foods and plan your meals wisely.

Fats for Energy Production

There are many different compounds that are found in the food we eat, as well as our bodies, that can be classified as *fats*. Besides water, fat is the second most abundant substance that the body is made of. Physiologically, there are three types of fats: triglycerides, phospholipids, and sterols. The triglycerides are what the majority of the fat that is found in the body and food is made of. The phospholipids—that consist of two fatty acids, a glycerol backbone, and a phosphate group—can be found in plants and animals and it's what the cell membranes of the tissues are made of. The sterols are different because they have carbon rings and not carbon chains. The most common sterol is cholesterol.

Dietary fat, although it is mostly blamed for weight gain and numerous health problems, is actually a nutrient that is essential for our overall health. The stored fat, also called adipose tissue, works as a cushion for our organs, it covers the nerves, it moves the vitamins throughout the body, and represent a huge reserve of stored energy. When we eat more calories than we should, we gain weight and store more fat within our bodies, which can open the door for many health complications.

Types of Fat

But not all fat will raise the bad cholesterol levels, and not all fats can harm us. Just like carbohydrates, all fats are also not created equally. There are three types of dietary fat:

Saturated Fat - this type of dietary fat is mainly found in animal sources such as red meat, dairy products, eggs, as well as commercially made cookies, cakes, and pies. The saturated fat is solid at room temperature, and it has been linked to some health problems. Because of that fact, it is wise to limit the amount of saturated fat to about 10 percent of the total calorie intake.

Unsaturated Fat - this type of fat can be classified into monounsaturated fat and polyunsaturated fat. The unsaturated fat is what we consider to be the 'good' type of fat, as it has been linked to health benefits such as lowering cholesterol and preventing the risk of cardiovascular diseases. The unsaturated fat is liquid at room temperature and can be found in avocados, fish, olive oil, canola oil, flaxseed, almonds, soybeans, fish, etc.

Trans Fat - the type of fat that nutritionists advise us to steer clear of. It is known that this 'bad' type of fat can increase the risk for heart disease, as well as increase the cholesterol levels. The trans-fat is made when the liquid unsaturated fat is turned into a solid and should be limited.

Providing the Energy

Do you know that a single gram of fat equals 9 calories? This, as well as our enormous ability to store fat within our bodies, make fat the largest energy reserve. A pound of stored fat can provide with 3,600 energy calories. And although these energy calories are not that accessible for quick and intense workouts such as weight lifting, they are absolutely essential for athletes that train with a long and slow intensity, such as endurance exercises like running, swimming, walking, or cycling.

Fat does not only provide the most important energy for fueling long exercises such as marathons or triathlons, but it is also necessary to access the stored energy from carbs during workouts with higher intensity.

There are a couple of factors that accessing the fuel from fat when exercising depends upon:

- It is slower to digest fat.

- It takes time to convert stored fat into energy, and this process can sometimes take up to 6 hours. In order to use it as fuel, the body first needs to break down the consumed fat completely, and then pass it to the working muscles.

- It takes a great amount of oxygen to convert fat into energy, which can only happen if the intensity of the workout is not that high and the athlete does not have trouble breathing.

That being said, it is of great importance that you, as an athlete, are mindful about how you consume fat. You need to be careful about the type of fat you consume, the amount of fat, as well as the timing. Generally, it is not recommended to eat fat during or right before a workout.

Protein for Energy Production

When it comes to the amount of protein you need to consume in order to boost your athletic performance, there are quite a lot of conflicting theories. And if you are a member of a gym and regularly spend some time on the track there, you know what I am talking about. You can hear the term protein shakes, egg whites, and meat, maybe too often. But wait... weren't meat, egg whites, and other saturated fats supposed to be limited to 10 percent of the daily calorie intake? Now you are confused, right? Well, the answer is quite simple. As we said, the backbone of your diet should be carb-rich foods such as veggies, grains, fruit, not meat. There is no need for you to eat giant stakes every night in order to strengthen your bones. You are not training to become a bodybuilder. In fact, even a bodybuilder's diet should mainly consist of carbohydrate-rich foods. If your diet lacks carbs and is high in protein, it will only provide poor fuel for the muscle contractions which can lead to poor performance and injuries.

If we are looking for the least important macronutrient for energy production, beyond doubt, protein is the one. However, that doesn't mean that you should ditch protein completely. The protein consumption of people that are physically active usually is not balanced. People either overindulge in protein-rich foods, for instance, bodybuilders, weight-lifters, etc., or they either switch it with salad instead. The truth is, neither the first nor the latter will provide adequate energy.

The Needs for Protein

Not everyone has the same needs for protein. Here is who needs protein the most:

- Endurance athletes—5 percent of their stored energy should come from protein. This is especially important if the blood sugar is low, or the stores of muscle glycogen exhausted.
- Dieters—those people that follow certain diets that lack the adequate amount of calories need extra protein since the protein they consume is mostly burned for energy and has no role in repairing the muscles.
- Teenage athletes—since protein is crucial for the growth and development of the muscles, growing teenage athlete should definitely include it in their diet.
- People with lower physical condition—those people that are not that physically active, are untrained, and are just starting an exercise program crave protein in order to build their muscles.

Here is how much protein is actually recommended:

Type of Person	Protein g per Each lb of Body Weight
Sedentary grown-ups	0.4
Recreational adult athletes	0.5—0.7
Endurance athletes, adult	0.6—0.7
Teenage athletes	0.7—0.9
A person that wants to build the muscle mass	0.7—0.8
Athletes that restrict calories	0.8—0.9
Average protein consumption for male endurance athletes	0.5—0.9
Average protein consumption for female endurance athletes	0.5—0.8

Now, see which one of the groups above you fall into. For instance, if you are an active female swimmer, then you fall under the 'endurance athletes, adult' category. The only thing you need to calculate the daily protein intake that is recommended for you is to know your scale weight. For instance, if it is 118 pounds, then you will need from 70.8 grams to 82.6 grams of protein per day.

118 lb x 0.6 g/lb = 70.8 grams of protein

118 lb x 0.7 g/lb = 82.6 grams of protein

Be Careful How Much Protein You Consume

Here is why you should be careful about the amount of protein you consume on a daily basis:

- If you overindulge on protein, you will not be able to use the stored energy from carbohydrates to fuel the muscle contractions.

- We know that protein breaks down into urea, which means that those people that consume protein excessively drink a lot of fluids, and go to the bathroom quite frequently. That frequent bathroom visits can be inconvenient during training and can negatively impact your performance.

- The diet that is high in protein is usually high in fat. Think bacon, juicy steaks, and fried eggs. If you want to keep your heart healthy and improve your performance, you should reduce the animal protein.

Protein for Vegetarians

Many athletes choose to avoid animal protein altogether. They don't eat meat, eggs, fish because they either consider it to be unethical, or they are either convinced that it is hard to digest and can bring numerous health-concerning issue. Whatever the reason one thing is sure, protein is an essential part of everyone's diet and a macronutrient that is needed during athletic performance.

The best way to ensure that their bodies will not lack protein is to replace the animal with plant-based protein. For instance, instead of meat, they should eat beans. Instead of dried fruits, they should eat dried fruits mixed with nuts. Instead of tomato spaghetti, they should eat tomato spaghetti with tofu.

The biggest illusion is that protein shakes and protein bars are the perfect meat substitute. Sure, they may be a good protein source, but they surely lack the nutrients that real and whole foods provide.

SUPERFOODS FOR ATHLETES AND PERFORMANCE

Many people assume that the athlete's diet is filled with grains and green veggies only, boring, and often tasteless. However, the properly balanced athlete's diet is flavorful, colorful and super-tasty.

Quality nutrition is the key to being able to push your limit, boost your performance, and achieve your athletic goals. Every endurance athlete who undergoes grueling exercises that are long, demanding, and often can take a toll on both the mind and body, should turn to nutrition when it comes to enduring the tough athletic challenges.

In order for you to be able to properly fuel the workouts, as well as recover afterward, it is of great importance that you fill your kitchen with these performance-boosting ingredients:

Chia Seeds. Since the Mayan and Aztec warriors consumed these tiny black seeds for power and endurance, people have definitely realized that chia seeds can indeed boost the performance without weighing you down during long exercises. They are a real nutrient dense ingredient that contains three times more antioxidants than blueberries and is rich in fiber, protein, iron, and calcium. Chia seeds also have hydrophilic properties due to their high amount of omega-3 fatty acids. That means that they can absorb more than 12 times of what they weigh in water, which will prolong the hydration. Besides that, these amazing black chia seeds also support the body regulation of other nutrients.

Walnuts. Walnuts are the perfect energizing snack on the go. Besides that they are yummy, they are also a plant-based protein that is rich in vitamin B, vitamin E, and loaded with antioxidants. The fact that they contain more omega 3-fatty acids of any other type of nuts tells us just how anti-inflammatory can this ingredient be. Walnuts will also keep your heart healthy, support bone health, lower the bad LDL cholesterol, and be a great support for your tough and demanding workouts.

Oatmeal. This heart healthy ingredient is a whole grain that is rich in complex carbs, as well as amazing fiber that can serve your body as a sponge that will absorb all of the fat and bad cholesterol from the bloodstream. Oatmeal has a low GI, and an amazing protein source which will provide a great energy release in the bloodstream which endurance athletes can really benefit from. Rich in minerals, vitamin B, and a number of antioxidants, oatmeal should be one of your top breakfast choices. The fact that it slows the glucose absorption means that oatmeal will curb your appetite and keep you energized for a longer period of time.

Canned Pumpkin. Now I know that the first thing that comes to your mind when you hear canned pumpkin (besides pumpkin pie) is sugar, but actually, a cup of canned pumpkin contains only 40 calories and 5 grams of fiber. A single serving of canned pie is three times your recommended Vitamin A intake. Canned pumpkin has an amazingly healthy blend of phytonutrients that your workouts can benefit from. Dump a cup of canned pumpkin with some low-sugar pumpkin pie ingredients and an energizing snack/desert.

Spinach. Seems like Popeye was right, although your muscles will not grow strong immediately after eating a can of spinach, but regular exercise, spinach is known to be one of the healthiest ingredients that contain a synergy of essential nutrients. Rich in antioxidants, beta-carotene, zeaxanthin, glutathione, folate, vitamin K, vitamin E...should I go on? The best part about spinach is that it is low in calories, 7 calories in a cup of spinach, so you can add it freely to your salads, omelets, smoothies, and meals, without being afraid that it will disrupt your daily intake.

Cherries. Cherries are one of the foods that are richest in antioxidants, and they will provide you with numerous health benefits, among which are better performance and quicker recovery for athletes. One research has shown that those runners that consumed raw cherry juice twice a day had less muscle pain after a long run. Another large study has concluded that cherries also lower the total weight, melt the body fat, beat inflammation, and with that, lower the risk for heart diseases.

Salmon. A healthy diet that lacks salmon is not healthy, period. Salmon is definitely one of the nutrient dense ingredients. This delicious fish is rich in vitamins B12 and B6, as well as omega 3-fatty acids which have proven to have astonishing results fighting inflammation, which athletes can really benefit from. Loaded with high-quality protein salmon is also great at repairing the muscles and offering a quick and painless post-workout recovery. The antioxidant called selenium found in salmon has shown to prevent the risk of heart diseases.

Cruciferous Veggies. Your mom was definitely right for forcing you to eat your broccoli. Cruciferous vegetables such as broccoli, kale, cauliflower, collard greens, and cabbage are packed with amazing nutrients and antioxidants that will help you prolong your endurance and heal your post-workout muscles faster. They are amazing sources of Vitamin C and vitamin K, and also rich in Vitamin A and folate. The best part about cruciferous veggies is the fact that they have more polyphenols than most of the vegetables and are loaded with anti-inflammatory properties that can minimize the risk of arthritis, muscle damage, as well as chronic pain.

Whole Grains. When they are unrefined, grains can pack you with an amazing fiber content, complex carbohydrates, as well as multiple minerals and vitamins. Because of their high content of amino acids, whole grains are also known to be a great fuel source that your performance can benefit from. Besides, they have a low GI, keep the blood sugar levels in check, as well as allow longer satiety.

Sweet Potato. This is probably the most delicious, versatile starchy veggie that you can use for chips, baked potatoes, soups, pies, pancakes, fries, and a number of other recipes. The most amazing thing about sweet potatoes is that they are packed with more beta-carotene than any other vegetable or fruit for that matter, and it is an amazing source of vitamins C, A, and E. They are great for removing radicals from the body, as well as lowering the blood pressure. Their high vitamin and mineral content make this sweet vegetable super beneficial for athletes, especially since sweet potatoes are rich in iron, potassium, copper, and manganese, which are all minerals that most athletes lack.

Eggs. Eggs that are rich in omega-3 fatty acids can pack athletes with riboflavin, B2, selenium, phosphorus, and of course, protein. Eggs high in omega 3 (such as Egglands Best) are an amazing source of BCAA (branched chain amino acid) leucine, which is the amino acid that is most important for muscles repair. Besides that, studies have shown that eggs have the tendency of increasing the good HDL and decreasing the bad LDL cholesterol.

Bananas. This is by far the most famous superfood for athletes, and the best pre and post workout snack. The reason why bananas are so popular among athletes is the fact that they can repack the body with the electrolytes that have been lost during the workout. Besides that, bananas are also amazing because of their high potassium and Vitamin B6 content, and the fact that they can regulate digestion and lower the blood sugar levels. After all, is there a more convenient snack?

Tomato Products. No, I don't mean just raw tomatoes, but tomato products like sauces as well. Why? Because, unlike most veggies, tomatoes are actually healthier when cooked. Sure, when heated, tomatoes tend to lose some of their Vitamin C content, however, the cooking process actually increases their antioxidant power which places cooked tomatoes on this ultimate performance superfood list. By adding tomatoes to your meals, you can optimize your performance, as well as the process of recovery faster.

Chocolate Milk. And you thought that only tasteless ingredients belonged on this list, right? Quit buying commercially prepared protein and carbohydrate beverages because a glass of chocolate milk is all it takes for you to enhance your recovery after a tough workout. In fact, chocolate milk has similar amino acid content like the commercial protein beverage, but with a 4:1 ratio of carbs to protein, which has been proven to ideal for post-workout muscle recovery. Packed with calcium, vitamin D, potassium, and sodium, chocolate milk is perhaps the tastiest, most inexpensive beverage to help you recover quickly.

Avocados. Is there really a diet or a meal plan that doesn't include avocados? I don't think so. Provide yourself with healthy, monounsaturated fats, and boost your athletic performance. Do you know that avocados contain 35percent more potassium than bananas? Besides, a single avocado can pack you with 20 different vitamins, phytonutrients, and minerals that your workout can really benefit from.

Lentils. Often called "the poor man's meat", legumes are an amazing source of fiber that can help you maintain your energy levels stable, as well as keep your blood sugar in check. High in protein and complex carbohydrates, it is safe to say that legumes will provide you with a long lasting energy and keep your muscles strong. Kidney beans, black beans, lentils, chickpeas, etc., are all great sources of protein and should be consumed regularly whether in soups, chilies, stews, or even salads and dips.

VITAMINS AND MINERALS

I have recently discovered that many athletes are mistaken that consuming more vitamins and minerals will improve their athletic performance. If you think so yourself, know that you are wrong. Neither vitamins nor minerals can directly impact your performance positively. They are not consumed in order to directly turn you into a better and fitter athlete. Vitamins and minerals do not provide with energy, however, they play a very important part in converting the food into energy.

And while consuming them regularly will not boost your performance, vitamin or mineral deficiency can surely result in poor performance. That is why it is of great importance that you make sure to pack your body with the essential vitamins and minerals.

Vitamin B1 (Thiamine)—Thiamine is important because it can help you break down the carbohydrates and protein that are essential for energy. The recommended daily intake is 1.2 mg for men and 1.1 mg for women. Just keep in mind that increasing the daily intake will not result in better performance. Great sources of Thiamine are whole grains and fortified cereals.

Vitamin B2 (Riboflavin)—Riboflavin is extremely important for the process of energy production, as well as for the formation of the red blood cells since it plays an important part in both processes. The recommended daily intake is 1.3 mg for men and 1.1 mg for women. Great sources of vitamin B2 are wheat germ, almonds, yogurt, milk, and fortified cereals and bread.

Niacin—Niacin is super useful since it supports both anaerobic and aerobic performance. The recommended daily intake is 16 mg for men and 14 mg for women. If you consume more or less than the recommended daily intake, your body's use of energy can easily shift from carbs to fat and the other way around, which can seriously affect the performance. Good sources of niacin are poultry, red meat, fish, enriched grain products, peanut butter, etc.

Vitamin B6 - This vitamin is super important for our overall health since it is involved in over 100 metabolic processes. What makes it especially essential for athletes is the fact that it is a part of the production of energy, as well as hemoglobin. The recommended daily intake of vitamin B6 is 1.3 mg for men that are 31 to 50 years old, 1.7 m for men that have 51 years or more, and 1.5 mg for women over 51 years. Sources of vitamin B6 are meat, eggs, fish, beans, oysters, seeds, and whole grains.

Vitamin B12 - Since it plays a huge part in the formation of the red blood cells, vitamin B12 is extremely important for getting enough oxygen to the tissues all over the body. You can see how consuming less of this vitamin than it is recommended can hurt the athletic performance, since an adequate amount of oxygen is crucial for enduring physical activities. The recommended daily intake is 2.4 mcg. Vitamin B12 is mostly found in animal products, so vegans and vegetarians should make sure to eat enough foods that are fortified with vitamin B12 to avoid becoming deficient.

Folate - Being essential for the production of cells, avoiding birth defects, as well as keeping the heart healthy, folate should be included in everyone's diet. The recommended daily intake is 400 mcg, and it is enough to support the requirements of energy that super active athletes have. Folate can be mostly found in dark leafy greens such as kale and spinach, whole grain breads, enriched grains, citrus fruit, and cereals.

Vitamin C - Being the most powerful antioxidant, Vitamin C can provide your overall health with a list of benefits. It is in charge of protecting the body from infections and cell damages, it is involved in the production of collagen—the thing that holds the muscles and bones together, it keeps the blood vessels and the walls of capillaries firm, it helps your body better absorb folate and iron, etc. It is extremely important for athletes not to consume less than the daily recommended intake of 90 m for men and 75 mg for women. As we know, Vitamin C is mostly found in citrus fruit, tomatoes, broccoli, sweet peppers, strawberries, and potatoes.

Panthothenic Acid - This is the vitamin that is especially important and helpful in the process of converting the carbs, fats, and protein into energy, which makes it pretty useful for athletes. The great thing is that pantothenic acid can be found pretty much everywhere, in both animal and plant products. Good sources include poultry, nuts, avocados, seafood, whole grains, etc. Try not to consume less than 5 mg of pantothenic acid a day to avoid hurting your performance.

Biotin - Playing a huge part in the process of energy production makes biotin an extremely important vitamin for those that are physically active on a regular basis such as endurance athletes. The daily recommended intake is 30 mcg, and good sources of biotin include eggs, fish, nuts, and soybeans.

Vitamin D - Although it is more of a hormone than a vitamin really, Vitamin D should be an inevitable part of athletes. It is mostly important for supporting the bone health which makes it essential for athletes that are involved in sports that are weight-sensitive such as cycling or running. The great part about Vitamin D is that you can pack your body with it even by exposing yourself to enough sunlight. Besides sunlight, amazing sources of Vitamin D are milk, cereals, eggs, seafood, and oil made of cod's liver. The daily recommended intake is 600 IU for people that are no older than 70 years, and 800 IU for those that have 71 years or more.

Iron - Essential for the formation of proteins that carry oxygen throughout the body, myoglobin, hemoglobin, as well as for many enzymes that are involved in energy production, iron is essential for endurance workouts since not having enough oxygen can negatively impact the performance. Most athletes tend to have low iron stores, so be sure to avoid this by consuming the recommended daily intake which is 18 mg for women and 8 mg for the average male. Remember, if you are vegan or vegetarian you will need to increase this daily intake to avoid iron depletion. Iron can be mostly found in red meat, seafood, beans, dried fruit, dark leafy greens, peas, fortified cereals, and bread, etc.

Calcium - Although we are all aware of the involvement of this mineral in the process of maintaining a proper bone health, calcium is also essential for proper muscle contraction. Although every human being needs to consume the recommended intake of calcium, for athletes this mineral is especially important since they tend to lose many minerals, calcium included, through perspiration. The recommended daily intake is 1,300 mg for teenagers and 1,000 mg for adults. Great sources of calcium include dairy products, spinach, collards, kale, okra, soybeans, white beans, fish, etc.

Zinc - Being a part of the process of producing energy, as well as playing an important role in building and repairing the muscle tissue, zinc is a mineral that can seriously hurt the athlete's performance if not consumed enough. The recommended daily intake of this mineral is 40 mg, and it can be mostly found in oysters, poultry, red meat, beans, whole grains, nuts, fortified cereals, and dairy products.

Magnesium - Being an important part in the cellular metabolism, proper hormonal functions, cardiovascular health, as well as regulating the neuromuscular and membrane stability, magnesium is pretty important for every active person. Endurance athletes should consume from 500 to 800 mg of magnesium a day, mostly by eating spinach, Swiss chard, pumpkin seeds, yogurt, almonds, black beans, etc.

Sodium - Being a critical electrolyte especially for those athletes that tend to sweat more, sodium should be a part of every athlete's diet since it is extremely important in regulating the body fluids. The daily recommended intake of sodium really depends on whether or not the person sweats excessively or not, but the general rule is that every athlete should consume about 1 gram of sodium per each hour of high-intensity workout. Natural sodium is mostly found in celery, milk, and beets.

Potassium - Important for keeping the electrolytes and fluids in balance, as well as regulating the nerve transmission, potassium is hugely important for every athlete. The general rule is that everyone older than 14 years should consume 4,700 mg of potassium a day, even athletes. Great sources are winter squash, sweet potatoes, potatoes, white beans, avocados, bananas, yogurt, etc.

SUPPLEMENTS FOR ENHANCING ENDURANCE PERFORMANCE

Probably the main questions that athletes ask dietitians are "Am I consuming enough vitamins and minerals?" and "Should I take any supplements?" And while no one can deny the fact that ingesting the adequate daily consumptions of minerals and vitamins through raw food, whole food is by far the best way to go, but not everyone can actually benefit from this. Take vegans and vegetarians, for instance, or people that are allergic to some types of food. Not being able to receive the necessary nutrients the right way means that it is time for a different approach.

Despite the fact that they are often backlashed by people, taking supplements when needed can be quite beneficial and will help you stay healthy. However, do not take these over-the-counter. Do regular blood tests and consult with your physician. You should take these supplements only if and when your doctor finds out that you are deficient of a certain micronutrient. If you are thinking about taking a certain supplement to boost your performance, run that idea by your physician first.

Creatine Monohydrate—Creatine supplementations has shown to be successful in reducing the recovery time, as well as improving the speed, power, and endurance during training sessions. The recommended dosage is 3 to 5 g a day.

Multivitamins—if you are vitamin deficient your doctor may suggest taking multivitamins to replace that deficiency and avoid poor performance. Although most people take multivitamins on their own, remember than most vitamins can hurt also hurt your workout of taken in greater dosage than what's recommended. Consult with your doctor first, before heading to the pharmacy.

BCAAs—BCAAs are important for hundreds of the bodily functions, and for athletes, they are essential for their recovery-enhancing effects, endurance-improving properties, as well as their ability to stimulate the protein synthesis. The doctors usually prescribe BCAAs when there is a lack of protein intake.

Fish Oil—if you consume less omega-3 fatty acids than recommended, then you should definitely think about supplementing with fish oil. Although it can be consumed through a number of other healthy ingredients such as walnuts, flaxseed, dark leafy greens, etc., your doctor may suggest taking omega 3 supplements if you are a vegetarian and don't eat fish. Another great omega 3 supplement is flaxseed oil.

Protein Powders—No, not every athlete should indulge in protein shakes, although most people believe the contrary. You are most likely to get enough protein through from your balanced diet, and if you consume a wide variety of protein-packed foods, there is surely no need for supplementing. However, if for some reason your diet lacks protein, taking supplements such as whey protein and casein protein may be the best option.

Glutamine—Being the most abundant amino acids in the body, you can only imagine how important glutamine must be for our overall health. You must be thinking, if it is so abundant, why supplement it, right? Well, the truth is, even though we have great stores of glutamine, athletes tend to drain the glutamine with their intense workouts. If glutamine stores are drained and not replenished, it can lead to muscle breakdown and some other serious injuries. If your doctor finds out that you have low levels of glutamine that can compromise your health, he or she may suggest taking 20 grams of glutamine supplement a day.

FLUIDS AND ELECTROLYTES

Do you know that when you are exercising your muscles actually generate twenty times more heat than when you are resting? That is why people sweat when active, to dissipate the heat. The sweat then evaporates and cools the skin, which then cools the blood, which cools the entire body. And since the more you exercise, the more you sweat, and the more water you lose, it is pretty obvious how hydration plays a huge part alongside your healthy diet in order to support your athletic performance and avoid injuries.

However, keeping yourself hydrated is easier said than done. Not all of us are made the same, and not all of us lose sweat the same way. Some people tend to sweat more than others and therefore need a higher water requirement. This chapter will help you learn how to stay hydrated and keep the water content in your body in check.

Up to 60 percent of the human body is water. That meant that a 150-pound man has approximately 10 to 12 gallons of water inside his body. Water is in charge for many different processes. It transports oxygen, glucose, and fats throughout the bloodstream and to the working muscles, as well as carries away byproducts such as carbon dioxide. In the urine, it is present to eliminate the waste products. In the sweat, it is there to dissipate the heat, regulate the temperature, and stop our bodies from cooking to death. It is also present in the saliva to help with food digestion. Water is also in charge of lubricating the joints and cushions the organs. In short, water means life.

You can see how losing too much water content through sweat and not replacing it on time can prevent the natural occurrence of these processes, which can not only lead to poor performance and fatigue, but also more serious injuries, and in some extreme situations, death.

Dehydration and Water Replacement

But like I said, everyone loses water through sweat differently, so the general rule of 8 glasses of water per day doesn't really apply to endurance athletes. Okay, so how to know if we consume enough water? You may think that the thirst is the greatest indicator that you are water deficient and should replenish, however, by the time that the warning signal that you are thirsty kicks you, you will already be pretty dehydrated, which by no means is good for your performance. The best way for you to check if you are doing a good job hydrating yourself is to weigh yourself before and after exercise. If you end your training session lighter than how you started is that can be a sign that you do not hydrate well. During exercise, you lose water, and if you end the session with fewer pounds that means that you haven't replaced the water loss.

Although the general rule for athletes is to drink 7 to 10 ounces of water in every 20 minutes of training, this doesn't really apply to everyone since the needed water consumption really depends on the entire metabolism, sweat rate exertion level, etc. The best indicator, however, is your scale. The numbers on your scale will show you if you need to lower or increase the amount of water you drink during a training session.

The Electrolytes

But sweat is not entirely made of water. The sweat you lose during exercise also contain electrically charged particles—electrolytes—that are important for keeping the water content in balance so it can regulate the natural processes within the body. Of course, the number of electrolytes you lose during exercise depends on how much you sweat, however, this is the general chart of the number of different electrolytes you lose in 2 pounds of sweat:

- *Sodium—800 mg*
- *Potassium 200 mg*
- *Calcium 20 mg*
- *Magnesium 10 mg*

That is why, instead of drinking only water, I suggest consuming fluids that also contain a little bit of salt (sodium) that will help stimulate the thirst, a little bit of potassium that will help you replace the loss of sweat and a little bit of carbohydrate for extra energy. Ideally, the beverage you will consume during exercise should contain about 100 to 170 mg of sodium per 8 ounces, 50 m of potassium per 8 ounces, and 10 to 24 grams of carbs per 8 ounces. Of course, if you do not like the idea of drinking anything other than plain water during exercise, you can always consume these nutrients via a balanced workout snack.

ENERGY TO FUEL

The food—or starches in particular—that we consume gets partially digested in our mouth by the saliva. After being swallowed, the food goes into the stomach, where it is liquefied with intestinal juices and then broken down into smaller particles. Then the food is emptied into the small intestine. There, starches are broken down into sugars, protein gets digested into amino acids, and the fat into fatty acids. The nutrients of the food now become available to our body. The small digestive products are transferred throughout the bloodstream to fuel the body. Digestive food components are also stored in the liver for future use. The indigestible products are transferred to the large intestine from where they are excreted.

And that is the process of how the energy we receive through the food can fuel our body. But when you are performing physically demanding activities where more fuel is needed, you need to know exactly when, what, and how much you should put in your mouth in order to receive the needed energy to endure the workout.

Fueling before Workouts

One of the biggest mistake and a real performance decreaser that most athletes are unaware of is the fact that they are more concerned with the reward, rather than with the pre-workout needed. And by reward I mean those cupcakes and candy bars you indulge in after a tough exercise in order to treat yourself for doing well. Instead of obsessing about the post workout treat, focus on the pre workout fuel.

Think of your body as a car. Just like your car needs fuel in order to transport you, the same your body needs fuel to perform and endure the physical activity. The fuel you need for athletic performance needs to be nutrient dense and contain the right amount of macronutrients. The fact that ditching food prior the exercise will result in more burned fat is only a myth since not fueling properly will have a counter effect on your performance.

Remember, your pre-workout meal has to be rich in carbs, contain adequate protein, and very little or no fat, if you are about to consume a meal not that long before the actual workout. For instance, if you are about to exercise early in the morning and you eat your breakfast 1 hour prior the workout (since, let's face it no one would get up in 3 or 4 AM in order to eat a proper breakfast), then you shouldn't load on fats since they cannot be digested within that time period. A fruit smoothie or a light yogurt and a piece of fruits are a great pre morning workout meal. After the training, you can enjoy a full meal within 2 hours post exercise.

Otherwise, you should always allow at least three or four hours for a full meal to properly digest before a workout. High-calorie meals take longer to digest than light snacks, so give your body the time. If you are afraid that that meal will not provide you with enough energy, have a half of banana 20 minutes before the workout for some extra potassium.

It is also of great importance to have a carb-rich dinner the night before, as well as to be properly hydrated. Another thing you should avoid eating before workouts is new food. Do not experiment with food prior the exercise but rely on familiar, safe choices to avoid upsetting your stomach and hurting your performance.

Fueling During Workouts

Just as it is important to fuel yourself before exercising, the same way it is important to stay fueled throughout the exercise. Unfortunately, our bodies do not work like your car's petrol tank. You cannot simply pack yourself with enough fuel to last you for tough and extensive exercises. That is why it is of great importance to ingest nutrients and energy sources during the exercise as well.

Those workouts that last longer than one hour should be balanced with enough fluids and carb to keep your energized. Choosing to consume about 100 to 250 calories of carbs after 60 minutes of training can have a serious positive impact on your stamina. And the best part of all is that your body doesn't care if you receive the fluid in a liquid or a solid form as long as it receives the essential nutrients. Whether it is better to snack on an energy bar while cycling or enjoy a sports drink loaded with carbs is entirely up to your own preferences. However, most people find mixing foods with fluids to be most convenient. That is why it is strongly suggested that instead of taking just a sports drink with you, you choose a sports drink that is mixed with banana or energy bar.

For moderate endurance workouts, the carbohydrates provide about half of the energy. Once you start exhausting the carbs from your muscles stores, you start depending on the blood sugar only. That is why it's super important to consume carbs during the exercise as well, because that way you provide your body with an extra source of energy.

Now, some athletes believe that consuming more carbs while exercising is better, but this is not true. If you choose to consume more food than your body can actually digest, you slow down the process when the fluids can leave your stomach and replace the loss of sweat. That means that if you choose to consume more carbs than needed, they will not only be useless to you, but they will also cause you intestinal distress. Unabsorbed carbs will just sit in your tummy, making it harder for your digestive organs to do their job efficiently. With that being said, no, more carbs do not mean more fuel. Our body is not a petrol tank. You cannot simply fill it all the way up and expect to use all of the consumed food for energy. It simply doesn't work that way.

Post-Workout Recovery

Post workout recovery is not about satisfying your taste buds, but your muscles. No, I do not mean that after extensive exercises you should dive into a bowl of tasteless and boring food, however, you definitely need to be mindful about the food you eat after workouts.

Proper nutrition is of great importance for the athletic recovery, so, remember this the next time you feel sore and stiff. A chocolate cake may please your tongue more than baked sweet potatoes, sure, but other than that it will not make you feel any better, and your muscles will still be stressed. However, your post workout meals shouldn't always be that boring. You can also enjoy a protein bar and a glass of chocolate milk post-work, which, let's face it, it is a lot yummier than sweet potatoes.

Another thing that you should be concerned about is to replenish the glycogen in your muscles, which is extremely important, if not crucial, if you have just finished a hard workout and you plan on exercising again after 6 hours. In that case, you will need to consume foods that are rich in carbs but also contain some protein for instance oatmeal or sweet potatoes. The target intake for such a recovery is 0.5 grams of carb per each pound of your weight, consumed in intervals of half an hour, for the next 4-5 hours.

For instance, if you are a 150-pound man, you should consume 150 x 0.5 = 75 grams of carbohydrates. And since 1 gram of carbs equals 4 calories, you will need approximately 300 calories from carbs consumed within the first hour after the workout.

Part II: The Ultimate Meal Plan for Endurance Athletes

If you are not that good at cooking, or preparing meals for that matter, then chances are you are still confused about what to eat even after the first part of this book has explained to you the basics of your sports nutrition. But don't worry, my guidance doesn't stop here. In this chapter, you will find a carefully created 4-week meal plan that will assist you on your athletic journey and show you what your performance-boosting meals should look like.

PLANNING WISELY

Although some will say that consuming 4-5 main meals and a couple of snacks a day is best, I don't see the point of that much cooking and meal prepping if you know how to carefully balance and plan three healthy meals and two filling snacks throughout the day. Besides, it is a lot more convenient to have three main meals assuming that you are also working and need time for demanding and extensive exercises.

Breakfast

They don't say that breakfast is the most important meal of the day for no reason. Skipping breakfast is perhaps the biggest crime you can make, so make sure not to do it. Avoid the clichés like "I don't have time to make breakfast", "I am running late for work", "I am not hungry" or "I am trying to lose weight", because neither one of these is a reason not to fill your tummy in the morning. Skipping breakfast can actually result in irregular eating patterns and will cause you to choose unhealthier snack choices which will not be good for your waist.

If you are not hungry in the morning that is only a sign that you have had way too many calories for dinner, so try to regulate that and start adapting a breakfast eating habit.

Your breakfast shouldn't be too heavy; just because we say it is the most important meal, it doesn't mean that it should be abundant, fatty, and juicy. Oatmeal, cereals, eggs, toast, pancakes, breakfast smoothies, bagel, etc., are all good breakfast choices. Don't forget to throw in some fruits, veggies, milk, and yogurt. A half of grapefruit is always welcome for breakfast.

Lunch

Although breakfast gives you the perfect energy kick in the morning, lunch is just an important. It gives provides you with the right nutrients to recover from the morning or noontime workouts, as well as pack you with the fuel for the afternoon exercises. And while the lunch is best consumed after noon, I say listen to your gut and eat by hunger, not by the clock. Those days when you will exercise more, you will be obviously hungrier than those with low-intensity workouts, so try not to wait for the afternoon snack hungry.

The best way to ensure that your lunch will be filling is to strive for at least 500 calories. That may include some meat, a pita bread, a salad, a fruit, some yogurt, or something similar to this. Dinner leftovers can also make yummy lunch.

If you have your lunch at work, try not to buy it but to pack your own lunch. That is the only way you can really keep track of exactly how much food—and of what quality—goes into your belly.

Snacks

I suggest two snacks—the first one between breakfast and lunch and the second one between lunch and dinner. Snacks should be convenient, simple, and shouldn't take long to prepare. They should provide you with enough energy and nutrients to keep you full until the main course.

Great snack choices are fruits with yogurt, popcorn, pretzels, smoothies, crackers, muffins, biscuits, veggies with dips and spreads, dried fruits, nuts, seeds, etc.

Dinner

As I said, dinners should be filling, but not too abundant. Otherwise, you will not be hungry in the morning, and the whole eating pattern will surely get disrupted. The key to cooking healthy and balanced dinners is purging the unhealthy food choices away, and stocking your kitchen with healthy ingredients.

When cooking dinner, choose at least three, if not all five food groups: grains, protein, fruits, vegetables, and dairy.

THE 4-WEEK MEAL PLAN

Below you will find a 4-week meal plan that your athletic performance can benefit from. The meal plan is healthy, balanced, and will provide you with the adequate nutrient intake to keep you healthy, support endurance and faster recovery. However, know that this meal plan is not set in stone. You can tweak it to your liking by adding and omitting ingredients as long as you follow the general guidelines from the first part of this book.

If you are training for a marathon or a triathlon, you will need a balanced meal plan for 12 weeks, not 4. You can easily take this meal plan as a base and shape the meal plan for the rest of the weeks according to this one. The point is to base your diet on carb-rich foods, lots of veggies, fruits, decent protein amount, dairy, nuts, grains, and seeds.

This meal plan does not include nutritional info for the sole reason that every single one of you should follow different nutritional guidelines. Make sure to calculate what your daily carb and calorie intake should be, and prepare these meals accordingly. For instance, if a dinner includes a cup of brown rice and your calorie intake won't allow it, reduce the amount but also reduce the amount of the other ingredients to keep the meal balanced.

The bottom line is to keep the right proportions and shape the meal plan according to your body's requirements.

WEEK 1

Day 1

Breakfast:

- 2 Hardboiled Eggs
- 2 slices of Whole Wheat Bread, toasted
- 2 tbsp. Cream Cheese
- ½ Tomato
- 1 glass of Orange Juice

Snack 1:

- ½ cup Popcorn
- ¾ cup Yogurt
- ½ cup mixed Fruit

Lunch:

- 1 serving White Asparagus Soup
- ½ Pita Bread
- 1 cup Green Salad
- 1 ounces of Cheese
- 1 Peach

Snack 2:

- 1 Banana
- 4 Whole Wheat Biscuits
- 1 cup Milk

Dinner:

- 1 Serving Polenta and Lamb Shanks
- 1 cup Sauteed Veggies
- 1 cup Pomegranate Juice

Day 2

Breakfast:

- 1 cup Oatmeal
- ¼ cup Blueberries
- ½ Banana
- 1 tbsp. Chia Seeds
- 1 glass of Apple Juice

Snack 1:

- 1 Whole Wheat Muffin
- ¾ cup Milk
- A handful of Walnuts

Lunch:

- 1 Fish Tacos
- ½ cup Yogurt
- 1 cup Green Grapes

Snack 2:

- 3 tbsp. crumbled Biscuits
- 2 tbsp. ground Almonds
- 1 cup Yogurt
- ½ cup diced Mango

Dinner:

- 4 ounces cooked Chicken
- 1 cup steamed Broccoli and Cauliflower Florets
- ½ cup Cherry Tomatoes
- 2 ounces of Cheese
- ½ cup Mashed Potatoes

Day 3

Breakfast:

- Avocado Salmon and Egg Toast
- ½ Grapefruit
- 1 glass Veggie Juice

Snack 1:

- 1 cup Milk
- A handful of Almonds
- 4 Biscuits

Lunch:

- 4 ounces cooked Turkey Meat
- ½ cup cooked Pasta
- ½ cup Steamed Veggies
- A handful of Baby Spinach
- 2 tbsp. Tomato Sauce

Snack 2:

- 1 ½ cup Fruit Smoothie
- 2 tbsp. Sunflower Seeds

Dinner:

- ½ cup cooked Peas
- 1 Sweet Potato, baked
- 2 ounces Tofu
- ½ cup sauteed Mushrooms
- 1 cup Cherries

Day 4

Breakfast:
- 1 cup cooked Millet
- 1 tbsp. Raisins
- 1 tbsp. dried Apricots
- 1 tbsp. Applesauce
- 1 cup Milk
- ½ Grapefruit

Snack 1:
- 1 slice of Whole Wheat Bread, toasted
- 1 tbsp. Peanut Butter
- ¼ Banana
- ½ cup Milk

Lunch:
- <u>Portobello Bruschetta</u>
- 1 cup Green Salad Mix
- 2 tbsp. Sour Cream
- 4 Baby Carrots
- 1 cup Fruit Juice

Snack 2:
- 1 cup Pretzels
- ½ cup Yogurt
- ½ cup Frozen Red Grapes

Dinner:
- 4 ounces ground Beef, cooked
- 1 cup Brown Rice
- ½ cup sauteed Veggies
- 3 tbsp. Tomato Sauce
- 4 tbsp. Shredded Cabbage
- 1 scoop of sugar-free and low-fat Ice Cream

Day 5

Breakfast:

- 2 scrambled Eggs
- 2 Whole Wheat Bread Slice
- 1 cup Mixed Veggies
- 1 ounce Cheese
- 1 Apple

Snack 1:

- 1 cup Milk
- A handful of Nuts
- A handful of Dried Fruit

Lunch:

- <u>Salmon Burgers</u>
- 1 Kiwi Fruit
- 1 Peach

Snack 2:

- 1 cup <u>Cinnamon Rice Pudding</u>

Dinner:

- 1 cup cooked Pasta
- 1 cup Sauteed Veggies
- 1 ounce Cheese
- 2 tbsp. Tomato Sauce
- 1 cup Yogurt

Day 6

Breakfast:

- 1 cup Raisin Bran
- 1 cup Milk
- ½ Banana

Snack 1:

- 1 cup Popcorn
- 1 cup Fruit Smoothie

Lunch:

- 1 cup Mashed Potatoes
- 4 ounces Fish Fillet
- 1 cup steamed Veggies
- ½ cup Baby Spinach

Snack 2:

- 1 cup Yogurt
- 1 Handful Nuts
- ½ cup Pineapple Chunks

Dinner:

- 1 serving Curry
- ½ Pita Bread
- 1 cup Green Salad Mix

Day 7

Breakfast:

- Egg and Rice Bowl
- ½ Grapefruit
- 1 Apple

Snack 1:

- A Handful of Sunflower Seeds
- 1 cup Green Grapes
- 1 ounce Cheese

Lunch:

- 1 Corn Tortilla
- 3 ounces cooked and shredded Turkey Meat
- 2 tbsp. Beans
- 1 tbsp. Guacamole
- ¼ Tomato
- ¼ cup Greens

Snack 2:

- <u>Lemon Strawberry Shortcake Trifle</u>

Dinner:

- 1 cup Yogurt
- 1 Chicken Drumstick
- ½ cup Sweet Potato, baked
- ½ cup Steamed Veggies
- ½ cup Raspberries

WEEK 2

Day 1

Breakfast:

- 1 Bagel
- 1 tbsp. Cream Cheese
- 2 ounces Smoked Salmon
- 1 cup Milk

Snack 1:

- 1 cup Fruit
- 1 cup Yogurt
- 1 tbsp. Raisins
- 1 tbsp. chopped Nuts

Lunch:

- [Winter Minestrone Soup](#)
- 1 Bread Slice
- 1 cup of Green Salad
- ½ Cucumber
- ½ Tomato

Snack 2:

- 1 tbsp. Peanut Butter
- 1 Banana
- 3 Biscuits

Dinner:

- 5 ounces Steak
- 1 cup Steamed Veggies
- ½ cup Mashed Potatoes
- 1 cup Cherries

Day 2

Breakfast:

- Coconut and Apple Breakfast Bowl
- ½ Grapefruit

Snack 1:

- 3 tbsp. Black Bean Hummus
- 1 Cucumber, cut into strips
- 1 Bell Pepper, cut into strips
- 1 Carrot, cut into strips

Lunch:

- 1 cup Clean Veggie Soup
- ½ Pita Bread
- 1 Peach
- ½ cup Yogurt

Snack 2:

- 1 Whole Wheat Muffin
- 1 cup Milk
- 1 tbsp. Peanut Butter

Dinner:

- ½ cup cooked Wild Rice
- ½ cup Sauteed Mushrooms
- 3 tbsp. White Sauce (made with heavy cream)
- 4 ounces cooked Chicken
- ½ cup Watermelon Chunks

Day 3

Breakfast:

- Vanilla and Blueberry Pancakes
- 1 cup Milk

Snack 1:

- 1 cup Fruit Smoothie
- A handful of Nuts

Lunch:

- Greek Quinoa Bowl
- 1 cup Yogurt
- A handful of Greens

Snack 2:

- 1 cup Cinnamon Rice Pudding

Dinner:

- ½ cup cooked Pasta
- 5 ounces Roasted Beef
- 1 cup Sauteed Veggies
- ½ Tomato
- 2/3 cup canned Pumpkin

Day 4

Breakfast:

- ½ Avocado
- ½ Tomato
- ½ cup of Yogurt
- 1 slice of Whole Wheat Bread, toasted
- 1 Poached Egg
- 1 ounce Cream Cheese
- ½ Grapefruit

Snack 1:

- 1 Protein Bar
- 1 cup of Milk

Lunch:

- 1 cup of Clean Chicken Soup
- ½ Pita Bread
- 1 cup of Green Salad
- 1 Apple

Snack 2:

- ½ cup canned Pumpkin
- A handful of Walnuts
- 4 tbsp. Pumpkin Seeds

Dinner:

- [Seafood Piccata](#)
- ½ cup Cherry Tomatoes
- 4 Asparagus Spears, steamed
- 1 Peach

Day 5:

Breakfast:

- 1 cup Oatmeal
- 2 tbsp. Shredded Coconut
- 2 tbsp. Chia Seeds
- 1 glass of Orange Juice

Snack 1:

- 1 cup Popcorn
- 1 cup Cherries

Lunch:

- [Pesto and Chicken Pita Pockets](#)
- 1 cup Melon Chunks
- ¾ cup Veggie Juice

Snack 2:

- 4 Biscuits
- 1 tbsp. Peanut Butter
- A handful of Almonds
- 1 cup of Milk

Dinner:

- 1 cup of cooked Brown Rice
- 1 cup of Sauteed Veggies
- 2 ounces Mozzarella Cheese
- ½ cup Frozen Yogurt

Day 6

Breakfast:

- <u>Polenta and Fried Egg</u>
- 1 Banana
- 1 glass of Apple Juice

Snack 1:

- 2 cup of Chocolate Milk
- A handful of Mixed Nuts
- 1 tbsp. Chia Seeds

Lunch:

- 2 slices of Whole Wheat Bread
- 2 ounces of Cheese
- 2 ounces of Grilled Mushrooms
- 1 cup of Pineapple Chunks

Snack 2:

- <u>Bacon and Blue Cheese Grilled Cabbage</u>
- 1 glass of Lemonade with a teaspoon of Honey in it

Dinner:

- 1 serving of <u>Beef Bourguignon</u>
- 1 cup Mashed Potatoes
- 1 glass of Orange Juice

Day 7

Breakfast:

- ½ Bagel
- 1 scrambled Egg
- 2 ounces of Sauteed Mushrooms
- 1 Bell Pepper, sauteed
- 1 tbsp. Cream Cheese
- A handful of Baby Spinach
- ½ cup Yogurt

Snack 1:

- 1 cup of mixed Berries
- 1 glass of Chocolate Milk
- 2 Vanilla Wafers

Lunch:

- Cheesy Squash and Sage Risotto
- 1 cup of Watermelon Juice

Snack 2:

- Tofu Lettuce Wraps
- 1 cup of Veggie Juice

Dinner:

- Chicken Stew
- 1 slice of Whole Wheat Bread
- A salad made with cucumber, tomato, peppers, and crumbled feta cheese
- 1 Peach

WEEK 3

Day 1

Breakfast:

- 3/4 cup Fiber-Fortified Cereal
- ½ cup Milk
- ½ Banana
- 2 tbsp. Blueberries
- 3 tbsp. ground Almonds

Snack 1:

- 1 cup of Pretzels
- 1 Tangerine
- 1 cup of Black Currant Juice

Lunch:

- 4 ounces of Chicken Meat
- 1 cup Sweet Potatoes Baked
- 1 ounce Mozzarella Cheese
- A handful of Kale drizzled with Balsamic Vinegar and Olive Oil
- ½ Tomato
- ½ cup Frozen Yogurt

Snack 2:

- 1 slice of Pumpkin Pie
- 1 cup of Milk

Dinner:

- <u>Sloppyless Joes</u>
- 1 cup of Fruit Juice by choice

Day 2

Breakfast:

- 1 Avocado
- 1 Whole Wheat Bread Slice, toasted
- 1 tbsp. of Hummus
- 2 Gouda Slices
- 1 slice of Lean Ham
- 1 cup of Orange Juice

Snack 1:

- 1 tbsp Cream Cheese
- ½ cup Yogurt
- ½ cup Strawberry Slices
- ½ Protein Bar, crumbled

Lunch:

- Kale and Farro Salad with Salmon
- 1 cup of lean Fruit Smoothie

Snack 2:

- 1 Whole Wheat Muffin
- 1 cup of Milk
- A handful of Nuts or a tablespoon of Peanut Butter

Dinner:

- 4-ounce Beef Steak, grilled
- 1 cup sauteed Veggies
- ½ cup Mashed Potatoes
- ½ cup shredded Beet with Olive Oil and Balsamic Vinegar
- 1 scoop of sugar-free and low-fat Ice Cream

Day 3

Breakfast:

- <u>Apple and Raisin Oatmeal Bowl</u>
- 1 cup of Milk
- ½ Grapefruit

Snack 1:

- 6 Crackers
- 4 Baby Carrots
- 3 tbsp. Hummus
- 6 Olives
- 1 Bell Pepper, cut into strips

Lunch:

- 1 cup of Chicken Noodle Soup
- 1 slice of Whole Wheat Bread
- 2 ounces Cheese
- ½ Tomato

Snack 2:

- A fruit salad made with 4 Strawberries, 1 Peach, ½ cup Pineapple Chunks, 2 tbsp. Blueberries, A handful of Blackberries, ¼ Apple, 2 tbsp. chopped Nuts

Dinner:

- <u>Shrimp Sandwich</u>
- 1 cup of Veggie Juice

Day 4:

Breakfast:

- 2 Pancakes
- 2 Bacon Slices
- 1 tbsp. Cream Cheese
- 1 Scrambled Egg
- 1 glass of Orange Juice

Snack 1:

- 4 Biscuits
- 1 tbsp. Fruit Jam
- 1 cup of Milk

Lunch:

- <u>Black Bean Soup</u>
- 1 cup of Green Salad
- 1 Pear
- 1 Lemonade with a teaspoon of honey

Snack 2:

- 1 cup Popcorn
- ½ cup Blackberries
- ½ cup Raspberries
- ½ cup of Apple Juice

Dinner:

- <u>Tuna Burger</u>
- 1 glass of Lime, Carrot, Orange, and Apple Juice
- ½ cup Frozen Red Grapes

Day 5

Breakfast:

- ¾ cup cooked Quinoa
- 1 tbsp. Chia Seeds
- 1 tbsp. Coconut Flakes
- 1 tbsp. dried Fruit
- 1 cup of Milk
- ½ Apple, grated

Snack 1:

- 1 <u>Nacho Cupcake</u>
- 1 cup of Fruit Juice

Lunch:

- 1 cup of Creamy Soup by choice
- 3 tbsp. Croutons
- 2 tbsp. Pumpkin Seeds
- 2 tsp Sour Cream
- 1 cup of Salad made with Leafy Greens, Cherry Tomatoes, Chickpeas, and 2 ounces of canned Tuna

Snack 2:

- 1 Smoothie made with Swiss Chards, Pineapple Chunks, Coconut Shavings, Coconut Milk, Lime Juice, Flaxseed and Banana

Dinner:

- 1 serving of <u>Pasta and Bean Skillet</u>
- 1 cup of Salad by Choice
- 1 Pear
- 1 cup of Cranberry Juice

Day 6

Breakfast:

- 2 slices of Whole Wheat Bread, toasted
- 2 tbsp. Butter
- 2 tbsp. Berry Jam
- 1 cup of Milk

Snack 1:

- ½ cup Pretzels
- 1 Orange Muesli

Lunch:

- Corn and Tomato Salad
- 1 cup of Clean Chicken Soup
- 1 Apple

Snack 2:

- 1 tbsp. Cream Cheese
- 1 ounce Blue Cheese
- A handful of Walnuts
- A handful of Grapes
- ½ cup Watermelon Chunks

Dinner:

- Goat Cheese Squash Pasta
- 1 cup Pineapple Chunks
- ½ cup Yogurt

Day 7

Breakfast:
- Breakfast Pizza
- ½ Grapefruit
- 1 glass of Apple Juice

Snack 1:
- 1 Apple
- 1 tbsp. Peanut Butter
- A handful of mixed Nuts

Lunch:
- ½ Pita Bread
- 1 ounces of Cheese
- 1/2 Tomato
- 4 ounces of Lean Beef, cooked
- A handful of Leafy Greens, wilted and drizzled with olive oil and balsamic vinegar
- ½ cup Broccoli Florets
- 1 Tangerine

Snack 2:
- 1 cup of Grilled Veggies
- 1 ounce of Mozzarella Cheese
- 1 glass of Pomegranate Juice

Dinner:
- 4-ounce Salmon fillet brushed with Dijon mustard, coated in chopped pistachios and baked
- 1 cup mashed Sweet Potatoes
- 4 Asparagus Spears
- 1 Carrot, cooked
- ½ cup Melon Chunks with ½ cup of Yogurt

WEEK 4

Day 1

Breakfast:

- 2 Pancakes
- 1 tbsp. Honey
- 3 tbsp. Yogurt
- 2 tbsp. Blueberries
- ½ Banana
- 3 Strawberries, sliced
- 1 tbsp. chopped Hazelnuts
- 1 cup of Milk

Snack 1:

- 1 Slice of Bread, toasted and cut into fourths
- 1 Tomato, sliced
- 2 ounces of Mozzarella Cheese

Lunch:

- 1 cup of Stew by choice
- 1 cup of Salad by choice
- ½ slice of Whole Wheat Bread
- 1 cup of Fruit Juice, by choice

Snack 2:

- 1 cup of Popcorn
- ½ cup of Homemade Raspberry and Lemon Frozen Yogurt

Dinner:

- 1 serving of <u>Cheese Spinach Cannelloni</u>
- 1 cup of Cherries

Day 2

Breakfast:

- Vegetarian Breakfast Taco
- 1 cup of Orange Juice
- 1 or ½ Pear depending on how big your tortilla is

Snack 1:

- 1 slice of Whole Wheat Bread, toasted, smeared with 1 tbsp of Peanut Butter, and topped with 4 Banana Slices
- ½ cup of Milk

Lunch:

- Raisin and Barley Salad
- 1 cup of Cantaloupe Chunks

Snack 2:

- ½ cup canned Pumpkin
- 1 tbsp. Whipped Cream
- A handful of Walnuts
- A glass of Apple Juice

Dinner:

- 6-ounce roasted Beef
- 1 cup of baked Root Veggies such as Potatoes, Carrots, Turnips, and Parsnips
- ½ cup of Cherry Tomatoes
- 1 ounce of Cheese
- 1 Peach

Day 3

Breakfast:
- 1 slice of Whole Wheat Bread, toasted
- 1 tbsp. Cream Cheese
- 2 slices of Lean Ham
- 1 scrambled Egg
- ½ Tomato, sliced
- ½ Banana
- 1 cup of Orange Juice

Snack 1:
- 1 Energy Sandwich Bomb
- ½ cup of Milk

Lunch:
- 1 cup of Clean Soup, Chicken or Veggie
- ½ cup of cooked Legumes
- 1 ounce of Cheese
- 3 ounces of flaked Salmon
- ½ slice of Bread

Snack 2:
- 3 tbsp. Hummus
- ½ Cucumber, cut into strips
- 1 Carrot, cut into strips
- 2 Celery stalks
- 1 glass of Apple Juice

Dinner:
- 1 serving of <u>Ratatoulie Spaghetti</u>
- 1 cup of Greek Yogurt
- 1 cup of Mixed Fruits

Day 4

Breakfast:

- 2 Egg, Spinach, and Feta Muffin Sandwiches
- 1 cup of Orange Juice

Snack 1:

- A handful of Nuts mixed with a Handful of Dried Fruit, 1 iced Mango, and ½ cup of Yogurt

Lunch:

- 1 Turkey Wrap
- 1 Peach
- 1 Tangerine

Snack 2:

- 1 cup of Chocolate Milk
- 1 Whole Wheat Muffin

Dinner:

- 1 cup of Lentil and Potato Dahl
- 1 cup of Salad by Choice
- 2 ounces of Cheese
- ½ slice of Whole Grain Bread

Day 5

Breakfast:

- 2 Waffles
- 1 cup of Favorite Fruits
- ½ cup of Yogurt
- 1 tbsp. Honey
- 1 tbsp. chopped Almonds

Snack 2:

- Caprese Salad made with 1 Tomato, 2 tbsp. chopped Basil Leaves, 2 ounces of Mozzarella Cheese, and drizzled with Olive Oil
- 1 Peach

Lunch:

- 4-ounces of Fish Fillet
- ½ cup of Mashed Potato
- ½ slice of Whole Wheat Bread
- ½ cup of steamed Cruciferous Veggies
- 1 Orange

Snack 2:

- 1 serving of favorite Pie, sugar-free
- 1 cup of Milk

Dinner:

- 1 cup Rice Noodles
- 1 cup Sautéed Veggies
- 1 ounce Tofu
- 1 cup Watermelon Chunks
- 4 Almonds

Day 6

Breakfast:

- 2 scrambled Eggs
- ½ Tomato
- 1 tbsp. Hummus
- 2 ounces sautéed Mushrooms
- 1 slice of Whole Wheat Bread
- 1 cup of Orange Juice

Snack 1:

- Almond and Cranberry Energy Bites
- 1 cup of Milk

Lunch:

- 1 cup of Baked Potatoes
- 2 tbsp. Beans
- 2 ounces Cheese
- A handful of Leafy Greens
- 1 cup of Red Grapes

Snack 2:

- A handful of Cashews
- 1 cup of Fruit Smoothie

Dinner:

- 1 serving of Beef Chile Relleno
- ½ cup of cooked Brown Rice
- 1 cup of Salad By Choice
- 2 Apricots

Day 7

Breakfast:

- 1 serving of Blueberry and Brioche Bread Pudding
- 1 cup of Milk

Snack 1:

- 1 cup of Baked Potato Chips
- 1 ounce Cheese
- ½ cup of Watermelon Chunks

Lunch:

- 1 Eggplant and Goat Cheese Sandwich
- 1 cup of Clean Veggie or Chicken Soup
- 1 Peach

Snack 2:

- 1 cup of Fruit Smoothie
- 1 cup of Popcorn

Dinner:

- 4-ounce of grilled lean Red Meat
- ½ cup of Brown Rice, cooked ½ cup of Mushrooms, sauteed
- 1 cup of Salad by choice
- ½ cup Yogurt mixed with ½ cup of favorite Fruit Chunks

Part III: Recipes for Athletic Performance

BREAKFAST

Egg and Rice Bowl

Serves: 1

Ingredients:

- 1 Egg
- ½ cup uncooked Brown Rice
- 1 tbsp. Soy Sauce
- 1 cup Water
- 2 tbsp. chopped Green Onions

Method:

1. Combine the rice and water in a pan over medium heat.
2. Cover the pan and let simmer for about 10 minutes.
3. As soon as it's cooked, immediately crack the egg into the bowl with hot rice.
4. Stir in the soy sauce.
5. Served topped with green onion slices.
6. Enjoy.

Vegetarian Breakfast Taco

Serves: 2

Ingredients:

- 1 small Sweet Potato
- 2 ounces Goat Cheese
- 4 small Flour Tortillas
- 4 Eggs
- 1 tbsp. plus 1 tsp Olive Oil
- 6 ounces Baby Spinach
- A Pinch of Salt

Method:

1. Heat one tablespoon of olive oil in a skillet over medium heat.
2. Dice the sweet potatoes and place them in the skillet. Saute for about 6 minutes, stirring frequently.
3. Meanwhile, place the spinach in another pan and heat them over medium heat until just wilted.
4. Beat the eggs and place them in the skillet with potatoes along with the remaining olive oil.
5. Stir and cook for a couple of minutes, to your liking.
6. Season with salt.
7. Divide the potato and egg mixture between the tortillas.
8. Top with spinach and crumbled goat cheese.
9. Serve and enjoy.

Avocado, Salmon, and Egg Toast

Serves: 1-2

Ingredients:

- 1 tsp White Vinegar
- Juice of ½ Lemon
- 2 Eggs
- 2 slices of Whole Wheat Bread
- 2 ounces of Smoked Salmon
- 1 Avocado, diced
- Salt, to taste

Method:

1. Fill a small pot with water and bring to a boil over medium heat.
2. Meanwhile, make an ice bath for the eggs.
3. Stir the vinegar in the boiling water.
4. Make whirlpool with a teaspoon at crack each egg at a time.
5. Let them cook for about 3 minutes; they should still be jiggly. After 3 minutes place them in the ice bath immediately.
6. Toast the bread slices in a toaster.
7. Combine the avocado with the lemon juice and some salt, and mash to make a paste.
8. Spread the avocado paste on the toasts.
9. Top with salmon and egg.
10. Serve and enjoy.

Apple and Raisin Oatmeal Bowl

Serves: 2

Ingredients:

- 1 tbsp. Brown Sugar
- 1 tbsp. Maple Sugar
- 1 cup of quick cooking Oats
- 1 small Apple
- ½ tbsp White Sugar
- ½ tbsp Vanilla Extract
- ½ cup Raisins
- ½ cup Milk
- 1 cup Water plus 2 tbsp. Pinch of Nutmeg, Pinch of Salt

Method:

1. Dice the apple and combine it with raisins, 2 tbsp. water, sugar, and all of the spices, in a pot.
2. Cover the pot and place it over medium heat to simmer.
3. Combine the oats, milk, and water, in another pot.
4. Stir in brown sugar, maple syrup, and salt.
5. Cook for about 5 minutes.
6. Combine the two mixtures together.
7. Divide between two bowls and enjoy.

Vanilla and Blueberry Pancakes

Serves: 2-3

Ingredients:

- 1 cup of Whole Wheat Flour
- 1 cup of low-fat Milk
- ½ tsp Salt
- 1 tbsp. low-fat Butter
- 1 cup of Blueberries
- 2 tsp Baking Powder
- 1 tsp Vanilla Extract
- 1 Egg

Method:

1. Combine all of the dry ingredients together in a bowl.
2. Gradually whisk in the milk.
3. Whisk in the egg and vanilla, making sure that there aren't any lumps left.
4. Heat a skillet over medium heat and place some of the butter in it.
5. Add about a 1/3 cup of the batter into the middle of the skillet, and then swirl the skillet to spread the batter evenly.
6. Cook for about two minutes on each side.
7. Repeat with the remaining batter.
8. Serve topped with blueberries and enjoy.

Egg, Spinach, and Feta Muffin Sandwich

Serves: 3

Ingredients:

- 6 English Muffins
- ½ Red Onion
- 6 Eggs
- ¼ cup plus 2 tbsp. Feta Cheese
- 1 Small Red Bell Pepper
- 16 ounces chopped Spinach
- 1 tsp Olive Oil
- Salt, to taste

Method:

1. Preheat your oven to 350 degrees F.
2. Heat the olive oil in a pan over medium heat.
3. Meanwhile, dice the veggies.
4. Place them in the pan and sauté for a couple of minutes or until soft.
5. Crack each egg into a ramekin.
6. Season with some salt, add eggs, spinach, and veggies.
7. Place the ramekins and muffins in the oven and bake for about 7 minutes.
8. Cut the muffins in half and assemble the sandwiches.
9. Serve and enjoy.

Blueberry and Brioche Bread Pudding

Serves: 4

Ingredients:

- 1 cup of Milk
- 2 Eggs
- 4 cups of Brioche Bread Cubes
- 1 tsp Vanilla Extract
- ½ cup of Sugar
- ½ pint of Blueberries
- Pinch of Salt

Method:

1. Preheat your oven to 350 degrees F.
2. Combine the bread and blueberries in a dish.
3. Combine the wet ingredients in a bowl, and pour the wet mixture over the bread and blueberries.
4. Stir to combine well.
5. Bake for about 45 minutes, or until golden and puffed up.
6. Serve and enjoy.

Polenta and Fried Egg

Serves: 2

Ingredients:

- 1 cup of Instant Polenta
- 1 tsp Butter
- 2 Eggs
- Pinch of Thyme
- 1 cup of Milk
- 1 cup of Water
- 1/2 Tomato, sliced
- ¼ cup grated Parmesan Cheese
- 1 tbsp. Olive Oil
- Salt, to taste

Method:

1. Preheat the oven to 350 degrees.
2. Drizzle the tomato with the olive oil and sprinkle with some thyme and salt.
3. Place in the oven until everything gets ready.
4. Heat a non-stick skillet over medium heat and add the eggs.
5. Season with some salt and cook until the desired consistency is reached.
6. Combine the milk and water in a pot and bring to a boil.
7. Add polenta and cook for about 3 minutes, stirring frequently.
8. Divide the polenta between two plates.
9. Top with eggs and tomato slices.
10. Serve and enjoy.

Breakfast Pizza

Serves: 2

Ingredients:

- 1 Bacon slice, cooked
- 1 small Pita Bread
- 1 cup Spinach, steamed
- 1 Egg
- ½ Tomato, sliced
- ¼ cup skim Ricotta Cheese
- Pinch of Nutmeg
- Salt, to taste

Method:

1. Preheat your oven to 350 degrees F.
2. Place the small pita in the oven and cook until crispy, about 10 minutes.
3. Meanwhile, fry the egg in a non-stick skillet over medium heat, to your liking; set aside.
4. Cook the bacon and drain the excess fat with a paper towel.
5. In a bowl, combine the spinach and ricotta.
6. Place the spinach and ricotta mixture on top of the pita bread.
7. Top with bacon and fried egg.
8. Season with some salt and nutmeg.
9. Serve and enjoy.

Coconut and Apple Breakfast Bowl

Serves: 1

Ingredients:

- 1 Apple, cored, peeled, and cut into chunks
- 3 tbsp. unsweetened shredded Coconut
- 2 Medjool Dates, pitted and chopped
- 1 tbsp. Almond Butter mixed
- 1 tbsp. of Water
- 3 tbsp. chopped Pecans

Method:

1. Place the apple, dates, pecans, and coconut in a food processor. Process until ground. Place the mixture in a bowl.
2. Combine the almond butter and water in a small microwave-safe bowl and microwave for 25 seconds.
3. Stir the almond mixture and drizzle it over the apple and cinnamon bowl.
4. Serve and enjoy.

LUNCH

White Asparagus Soup

Serves: 6

Ingredients:

- 2 pounds of Asparagus
- Juice of ½ Lemon
- 1 Shallot, diced
- 1 tsp Olive Oil
- 2 tbsp. Butter
- 4 Tarragon Sprigs
- ½ cup Heavy Cream
- 1 quart Vegetable Stock
- 2 tbsp. Flour
- ¾ cup White Wine
- 1 Garlic Clove, minced
- Salt, to taste

Method:

1. Heat the olive oil in a large pot over medium heat.
2. Add the shallot and cook for about 3 minutes.
3. Add the garlic and sauté for an additional minute.
4. Add asparagus, lemon juice, tarragon, stock, and season with some salt.
5. Bring the mixture to a simmer.
6. Cover the pot and let cook for 45 minutes.
7. Remove the tarragon and blend the mixture with a hand blender.
8. Melt the butter in a skillet over medium heat.
9. Add flour and whisk for a few minutes.
10. Gradually add the heavy cream.
11. Whisk the white sauce into the blended soup.
12. Bring the soup to a boil and remove from heat immediately.
13. Serve and enjoy.

Corn and Tomato Salad with Peppers, Feta, and Onion

Serves: 2

Ingredients:

- 2 Ears of Corn
- ¼ small Red Onion
- 18/4 cup crumbled Feta Cheese
- 3 Ripe Tomatoes
- 1 tsp Olive Oil
- ½ Red Bell Pepper
- ¼ cup chopped herbs
- 1 tbsp. Red Wine Vinegar
- Salt, to taste

Method:

1. Preheat your grill on high and grill the corn for about 8 minutes, until slightly charred.
2. Slice the peppers and onion, cut the tomatoes into quarters, and chop the herbs finely.
3. Let the corn cool a little bit before cutting the kernels.
4. Lace all of the ingredients in a bowl and mix to incorporate them well.
5. Serve and enjoy.

Cheesy Squash and Sage Risotto

Serves: 2

Ingredients:

- 1 ½ pounds Butternut Squash
- 1 tbsp. Butter
- 1 Garlic Clove, minced
- 1 ¾ cup Chicken Broth
- ½ cup of Brown Rice
- 1 ounce Goat Cheese
- 1/8 cup Grated Parmesan Cheese
- ¼ cup Dry White Wine
- ½ cup Water
- ½ Onion, chopped
- 1 tbsp. chopped Fresh Sage
- 1 tbsp. Olive Oil

Method:

1. Preheat your oven to 400 degrees F.
2. Peel and cut the squash lengthwise. Discard the seeds.
3. Place one half of the squash on a lined baking sheet and bake in the oven for about 15 minutes.
4. The other half cut it into small chunks.
5. When cool enough to handle, scoop out the flesh, and chop.
6. Heat the olive oil in a saucepan over medium heat.
7. Cook the onions for a couple of minutes.
8. Add garlic and cook for one more minute.
9. Stir in all the remaining ingredients (including baked and raw squash), except the sage, parmesan, and goat cheese.
10. Let it cook for about 18 minutes.
11. Finally, stir in the sage and the cheeses.
12. Divide the risotto between two bowls.
13. Serve and enjoy.

Salmon Burgers

Serves: 4

Ingredients:

- 1 ¼ pound Salmon
- ¼ cup chopped Red Onion
- 1 tbsp. Olive Oil
- 4 Buns
- 4 Lettuce Leaves
- ¼ cup chopped Red Onion
- 8 Tomato Slices
- 1 tsp Dijon Mustard
- 2 tbsp. Capers
- ½ cup Bread Crumbs
- ¼ cup Mayonnaise
- 1 Garlic Clove, minced
- 2 tsp Lemon Juice
- ¼ cup chopped Herbs

Method:

1. Cut the salmon into pieces and place it in a food processor.
2. Add capers, red onion, mustard, and 1 tsp lemon juice.
3. Pulse a couple of times until ground.
4. Stir in bread crumbs.
5. Make four patties out of the mixture.
6. Preheat your grill to high.
7. Add the patties and grill for about three or four minutes per side.
8. Combine mayo, herbs, garlic and lemon juice.
9. Add a lettuce leave on each bun and top with the salmon Pattie.
10. Spread the mayo mixture over the salmon patties and top with tomato slices.
11. Serve and enjoy.

Lentil and Spinach Salad

Serves: 4

Ingredients:

- 1 cup Green Lentils
- 3 Carrots
- 2 Celery Sticks
- 1 Garlic Clove
- 4 cups Water
- 16 ounces of Spinach
- 1 Small Fennel
- 1 small Yellow Onion, chopped
- ½ tbsp. Dijon Mustard
- 2 tbsp. Olive Oil
- 1 tsp Red Wine Vinegar
- Salt, to taste

Preparation:

1. Combine the lentils and water in a pot over medium heat, and bring to a boil.
2. Peel the onion and add it in the water
3. Chop one carrot and one celery stick and add them to the lentils.
4. Meanwhile, chop the remaining celery and carrots.
5. Heat half of olive oil in a Dutch oven and sauté the carrots and celery.
6. Discard the onion and drain the lentils. Transfer to a bowl.
7. Stir in the remaining veggies.
8. Stir in the remaining olive oil, mustard, vinegar, and some salt.
9. Mix to combine well.
10. Serve and enjoy.

Winter Minestrone Soup

Serves: 6

Ingredients:

- 2 Carrots
- 1 Potato
- 2 Garlic Cloves
- 1 small Head of Cabbage
- 16 ounces Spinach
- 1 Yellow Onion
- 15 ounces Cannellini Beans
- 1 tbsp. Olive Oil
- 4 sprigs Thyme
- 1 Bay Leaf
- 1 cup dried Macaroni
- 6 cups Vegetable Stock
- 1 sprig Rosemary
- 1 Celery Stalk
- Salt, to taste
- Parmesan Cheese, to taste

Method:

1. Dice the veggies.
2. Heat the olive oil in a large and heavy bottomed pan.
3. Add celery, onion, and carrots, and season with some salt.
4. Cook until soft for a couple of minutes.
5. Add garlic and cook for one more minute.
6. Add chopped cabbage, season with some salt and cook for 5 minutes.
7. Stir in beans, stock, and tomatoes.
8. Add the herbs and some more salt.
9. Let simmer for about 30 minutes.
10. Add the pasta and cook for as long as stated on the package.
11. Remove from heat.
12. Add spinach and some parmesan cheese.
13. Serve and enjoy.

Fish Tacos

Serves: 4

Ingredients:

- 16 ounces White Fish
- 2 tbsp. Blackening Seasoning
- 1 tsp Salt
- 1 tsp Olive Oil
- 4 Tortillas

Coleslaw

- ½ head Cabbage, sliced
- ¼ cup Sour Cream
- 1 tsp Honey
- ¼ Red Onion, sliced
- 2 tbsp. chopped Cilantro
- ¼ cup Apple Cider Vinegar

Salsa

- 1 Ripe Mango
- 1 tsp Honey
- ¼ cup chopped Cilantro
- ¼ small Red Onion
- ¼ Red Bell Pepper
- ½ small Jalapeno

Method:

1. Combine all of the slaw ingredients in a bowl and set them aside.
2. Dice the salsa veggies and mango and combine them in a bowl along with the rest of the salsa ingredients.
3. Heat the olive oil in a skillet over medium heat.
4. Cut the fish into pieces, season with salt and seasoning, and cook for about 5 minutes.
5. Place the slow on the bottom of the tortillas, then top with fish and salsa.
6. Serve and enjoy.

Kale and Farro Salad with Baked Salmon

Serves: 2

Ingredients:

- 1 cup dry Farro, soaked for 8 hours
- 6 Large Kale Leaves, torn into pieces
- 2 6-ounce Salmon Fillets
- ½ Onion, sliced
- ½ cup Shaved Parmesan Cheese
- ¼ cup Pumpkin Seeds
- 2 tbsp. Olive Oil

Dressing

- 2 tbsp. Lemon Juice
- 2 tbsp. Olive Oil
- 1 Garlic Clove, minced
- ¼ tsp Pepper
- ¼ tsp Salt

Method:

1. Rinse and drain farro.
2. Place it in a pan and cover with water.
3. Bring to a boil over medium heat. Reduce the heat to low and let simmer for 20 minutes.
4. Place the salmon fillet on a baking sheet and drizzle with 1 tbsp. olive oil.
5. Bake at 425 degrees F, for about 8 minutes.
6. Heat 1 tbsp. of olive oil in a skillet over medium heat.
7. Add kale and cook until it begins to char.
8. Place onion and cook until slightly charred.
9. In a large bowl combine the farro, charred kale, charred onion, parmesan, and pumpkin seeds.
10. Combine the dressing ingredients and drizzle the dressing over the salad.
11. Divide the salad between two bowls.
12. Top with salmon fillets and enjoy.

Portobello Bruschetta

Serves: 2

Ingredients:

- 4 Large Portobello Mushrooms
- 2 Pints of Cherry Tomatoes, sliced
- ¼ cup chopped Red Onion
- 3 Garlic Cloves, minced
- 2 tbsp. Balsamic Vinegar
- A handful of Basil, chopped
- 1 ½ cup small Mozzarella Bowls
- 1 tbsp. Olive Oil
- Salt, to taste

Method:

1. Preheat the grill to medium heat.
2. Place all of the ingredients, except the mushrooms, in a bowl and stir to combine them well.
3. Divide the mixture between the mushrooms.
4. Place the mushrooms on the grill, close the lid and cook for 10 to 15 minutes.
5. Serve and enjoy.

Turkey Wrap with Avocado Cream

Serves: 2

Ingredients:

- ½ Ripe Avocado
- 3 tbsp. Low-Fat Yogurt
- 2 Whole Grain Tortillas
- 4 ounces cooked and sliced Turkey
- 1 Large Tomato, sliced
- 2 Handfuls of Lettuce Leaves
- 2 tsp Lemon Juice
- Pinch of Salt and Pepper

Method:

1. Place the avocado, lemon juice, yogurt, salt, and pepper, in a food processor and pulse until smooth.
2. Spread the avocado cream on both tortillas evenly.
3. Top with turkey and tomato slices.
4. Arrange the lettuce leaves on top.
5. Roll the tortillas and cut them in half.
6. Serve and enjoy.

Greek Quinoa Bowls

Serves: 2

Ingredients:

- 1 cup Quinoa
- 1 ½ cups Water
- 2 ½ tbsp. apple Cider Vinegar
- 1 ½ tbsp. fresh Parsley
- 1 cup chopped Green Bell Pepper
- 1 cup chopped Red Bell Pepper
- ¼ cup Olive Oil
- 1/3 cup crumbled Feta Cheese
- 1 Pita Bread, cut into wedges
- Salt and Pepper, to taste

Method:

1. Rinse and drain the quinoa.
2. Combine it with the water in a pot over medium heat.
3. Cook until 15 minutes, or until fluffy.
4. Meanwhile place all of the other ingredients, except the pita bread, in a large bowl.
5. Let quinoa cook slightly.
6. Add it to the bowl.
7. Stir to combine the ingredients well.
8. Divide the quinoa salad between two bowls.
9. Serve with pita wedges and enjoy.

Eggplant and Goat Cheese Sandwich

Serves: 2

Ingredients:

- 1 Eggplant
- 1 tbsp. Goat Cheese
- 2 tbsp. Ricotta Cheese
- ½ Red Bell Pepper
- 1 tbsp. Olive Oil
- 2 Burger Buns
- 1 small Tomato, sliced
- 4 Red Onion Slices
- Salt, to taste

Method:

1. Preheat your grill to high heat.
2. Slice the eggplant into 1/3-inch slices and place it in a bowl.
3. Add bell pepper, olive oil, and some salt, and mix to combine.
4. Place them on the grill and cook for about 5 minutes on each side.
5. Combine the goat cheese and ricotta in a small bowl.
6. Spread the cheese evenly between the two buns.
7. Add grilled eggplant and pepper.
8. Top with tomato and onion slices.
9. Close the bun, press it, and grill on both sides for about a minute.
10. Serve and enjoy.

Spicy Raisin and Barley Salad

Serves: 4

Ingredients:

- 1 cup dry Barley
- 1 tbsp. Olive Oil
- 1 Garlic Clove, minced
- ¼ cup Pine Nuts
- ¼ cup Raisins
- 1 cup Vegetable Broth
- 1 Bell Pepper, diced
- 1 cup Water
- 1 can Navy Beans, rinsed and drained
- ½ tsp Turmeric
- ¼ tsp Cumin
- ¼ tsp Ginger Powder
- ¼ tsp Curry Powder
- ¼ tsp Cinnamon
- ¼ tsp Black Pepper

Method:

1. Combine barley, water, and broth, in a pan over medium heat.
2. Bring to a boil, reduce the heat, and let simmer for 20 minutes or until fluffy.
3. Heat the olive oil in a large skillet.
4. Combine the remaining ingredients in the skillet and cook for about 3 minutes.
5. Add the barley.
6. Stir until well combined.
7. Serve the salad warm and enjoy.

Black Bean Soup

Serves: 6

Ingredients:

- 1 cup chopped Onion
- 1 pound dried Black Beans
- 1 tsp Liquid Smoke
- 1 cup chopped Red Bell Pepper
- 2 tbsp. Olive Oil
- 3 Garlic Cloves, minced
- 3 cups Beef Broth
- ¼ cup Apple Cider
- 1 ½ tsp Cumin
- 1 ½ tsp Oregano
- 3 cups Water
- 1 Tomato, chopped

Method:

1. Place the beans in your Dutch oven.
2. Cover with water and place over medium heat.
3. Bring to a boil and let boil for about 2 minutes.
4. Remove from heat.
5. Cover the beans and let sit for about an hour.
6. Drain the liquid and reserve the beans.
7. Heat the olive oil over medium heat in the same Dutch oven.
8. Add onion and cook until soft for about 5 minutes.
9. Add garlic and cook for one more minute.
10. Add the remaining ingredients and stir to combine.
11. Bring to a boil and let boil for about 2 minutes.
12. Reduce the heat to low, cover the Dutch, and simmer for 2 hours.
13. Blend the soup with a hand blender until smooth.
14. Serve and enjoy.

Pesto and Chicken Pita Pockets

Serves: 2-4

Ingredients:

- 2 Chicken Breasts, boneless and skinless
- ¼ cup Pesto Sauce
- 1 tbsp. Olive Oil
- 6 cups mixed Vegetables cut into chunks (Bell Peppers, Zucchini, Red Onion)
- 1 tbsp. Olive Oil
- 2 Pita Breads
- Salt and Pepper, to taste

Method:

1. Preheat your oven to 425 degrees F.
2. Brush the chicken breast with ½ tbsp. olive oil and sprinkle with some salt and pepper.
3. Place the chicken in a baking dish.
4. Place the veggies in another baking dish and toss them with the remaining olive oil and some salt and pepper.
5. Place both pans in the oven and roast for about 10 minutes.
6. Flip everything and bring back to the oven. Cook the veggies for 10 minutes and the chicken for 15 more minutes.
7. Place them all in a large bowl, add pesto and stir to combine well.
8. Cut the pita breads in half and open the pockets.
9. Divide the chicken and veggie mixture between the pockets.
10. Serve and enjoy.

DINNER

Sloppyless Joes

Serves: 4

Ingredients:

- 1 pound ground Beef Meat
- 1 Carrot, grated
- 1 tbsp. Athlete Food Green Seasoning
- 1/3 cup Water
- 1 tbsp. Molasses
- 1 tbsp. Cane Sugar
- 2 handfuls of Baby Spinach
- 1 tsp Dijon Mustard
- ½ cup Ketchup
- 4 Buns
- ¼ tsp Chili Powder
- ½ tsp Oregano
- Salt and Pepper, to taste

Method:

1. Place the meat, seasoning, spinach, and carrot in a pan over medium heat.
2. Stir in the remaining ingredients (except the buns), and cook for 3 to 4 minutes.
3. Cut the buns open and divide the beef mixture between them.
4. Serve and enjoy.

Goat Cheese Butternut Squash Pasta

Serves: 2

Ingredients:

- 6 ounces of Farfalle Pasta
- 2 ounces Goat Cheese
- 2 cups diced Squash
- 2 tbsp. chopped Fresh Basil
- 1 tbsp. Olive Oil
- Salt, to taste

Method:

1. Fill two pots with water, place them over medium heat and bring them both to a boil.
2. Add a pinch of salt in both pots.
3. In one, cook the farfalle according to the package's instruction.
4. In the other pot, add the squash and cook it until soft (a fork can easily run through).
5. Drain the pasta and reserve 14/4 cup of the cooking liquid.
6. Add the olive oil to the pasta and toss to combine.
7. Bring the pasta back to the pot, add the reserved cooking liquid, butternut squash, chopped basil, and crumbled goat cheese.
8. Toss to combine well.
9. Serve and enjoy.

Slow Cooked Curry

Serves: 4

Ingredients:

- 1 ½ pounds boneless and skinless Chicken Thighs
- 2 Garlic Cloves
- 1 tsp Cumin
- 1 cup Half and Half
- 1 Jalapeno
- 8 ounces Tomato Paste
- 1 small Yellow Onion
- 1 tbsp. Olive Oil
- ½ cup Chicken Stock
- 2 tbsp. Butter
- 1 tsp Garam Masala Powder
- 1 ½ tsp ground Ginger
- Salt, to taste

Method:

1. Heat the slow cooker on high.
2. Slice the onion, heat the olive oil inside the slow cooker, and add the onion.
3. Mince the ginger and garlic and add them to the slow cooker.
4. Sauté for a couple of minutes.
5. Add the thighs.
6. Stir in the rest of the ingredients, except the butter and garam masala.
7. Set the slow cooker on low.
8. Close the lid and cook for about 4 hours.
9. Stir in the butter and garam masala.
10. Serve and enjoy.

Shrimp Sandwich

Serves: 2

Ingredients:

- 1 cup Shredded Cabbage
- 4 Onion Slices
- 12-inch French Baguette
- 12 large Shrimp
- 1 ½ tbsp. Ketchup
- 1 tsp Olive Oil
- 1 tsp Blackened Seasoning
- 2 ½ tbsp. Mayonnaise
- 1 tsp Lemon Juice
- 1 tbsp. Sweet Relish
- A pinch of Salt
- 1 cup shredded Romaine Lettuce

Method:

1. Preheat your grill to high.
2. Coat the shrimp with the olive oil and seasoning, in a bowl.
3. To make the sauce, combine the relish, ketchup, mayonnaise, lemon juice, and salt.
4. Grill the shrimp for a couple of minutes on both sides.
5. Cut the baguette in half and cut the halves open.
6. Spread half of the sauce on each baguette.
7. Add the onion slices, cabbage, and romaine.
8. Top with the shrimp.
9. Serve and enjoy.

Polenta and Lamb Shanks

Serves: 4

Ingredients:

- 4 Lamb Shanks
- 2 tbsp. Olive Oil
- ½ Onion
- 2 cups Marsala
- 28 ounces crushed Tomatoes
- 4 Pepperoncini, drained and chopped
- ¼ cup Tomato Sauce
- tbsp. Sugar
- 3 Thyme Sprigs
- 2 Bay Leaves
- 1 tsp Oregano
- 1 tbsp. Butter
- 1 tbsp. Sugar
- 4 cups of Water
- 1 cup of Polenta
- ½ cup grated Parmesan
- 1 tsp dried Oregano
- Salt, to taste

Method:

1. Preheat your oven to 350 degrees F.
2. Heat the olive oil in a large pan over medium heat.
3. Sprinkle some salt over the lamb shanks and cook them for about 5 minutes on both sides.
4. Meanwhile, chop all the veggies.
5. Remove the lamb from the pan and add the veggies.
6. Saute them for 5 minutes.
7. Stir in the tomato paste, marsala, herbs, tomatoes, and the lamb shanks.
8. Season with some more salt.
9. Cover the pan, place it in the oven, and bake for about 2 hours.
10. Fill a pot with 4 cups of water, and bring to a boil over medium heat.
11. Add polenta and cook for a couple of minutes, stirring constantly.
12. As soon as it starts thickening, stir in some salt, butter, and parmesan.
13. Divide the polenta among 4 plates.
14. Top with a lamb shank and some of the sauce.
15. Serve and enjoy.

Seafood Piccata

Serves: 2

Ingredients:

- ¼ cup White Wince
- 1 Garlic Clove, minced
- 2 tbsp. Parmesan Cheese
- Juice of 1 Lemon
- ¼ cup Flour
- 2 tbsp. Capers
- 1 tsp Olive Oil
- 2 4-ounces Fish Fillets
- 1 tbsp. Butter
- 4 ounces Angel Hair Paste
- 2 tbsp. chopped Parsley
- Salt and Pepper, to taste

Method:

1. Fill a large pot with water and bring it to a boil over medium heat.
2. Add the pasta and cook according to food instructions.
3. Rinse, drain, and divide between two plates.
4. Heat the olive oil in a large non-stick skillet over medium heat.
5. Sprinkle the fish with some salt and coat it with flour.
6. Place in the skillet and cook for a couple of minutes on each side.
7. Add the minced garlic and cook for about a minute to make the fish more fragrant.
8. Add the wine and let simmer for one minute.
9. Add the butter and parmesan cheese and cook for 10 seconds.
10. Divide the fish and sauce between the plates with pasta.
11. Serve and enjoy.

Winter Chicken Stew

Serves: 8

Ingredients:

- 3 Leeks, sliced
- 1 tbsp. Thyme
- 1 Onion, chopped
- 1 tbsp. Olive Oil
- 16 Chicken Thighs
- 1 Potato, grated
- 4 Garlic Cloves, sliced
- 6 cups Chicken Stock
- 2 tbsp. Rosemary
- 6 Carrots, chopped
- 2 Parsnips, chopped

Method:

1. Heat the olive oil in a large pot over medium heat.
2. Sauté the onions for a couple of minutes.
3. Add the garlic and cook for one more.
4. Add the stock, potato, rosemary, and thyme.
5. Add the chicken.
6. Bring the mixture to a boil.
7. Add carrots, leeks, and parsnips.
8. Cover the pot, reduce the heat, and let simmer for 40 minutes.
9. Serve as desired and enjoy.

Ahi Tuna Burger

Serves: 2

Ingredients:

- ¼ cup sliced Onion
- 2 tbsp. Mayonnaise
- 1 Avocado, sliced
- 2 4-ounce Ahi Tuna Fillets
- 1 ½ cups Shredded Cabbage
- 1 tbsp. Honey
- 1 tbsp. Sesame Oil
- 1 ½ tbsp. Rice Wine Vinegar
- 1 tbsp. Sriracha
- 1 tsp Olive Oil
- 2 Buns
- Salt and Pepper, to taste

Method:

1. Combine the cabbage, sesame oil, onion, honey, vinegar, and some salt and pepper, in a large bowl. Set aside.
2. Combine the mayonnaise with sriracha, and season with some salt and pepper.
3. Heat the olive oil in a pan over medium heat.
4. Season the tuna fillets with some salt and pepper, and cook them for about 1 minute on both sides.
5. Spread the mayo/sriracha mixture first, arrange the avocado slices second, top with the tuna fillets, and then add the coleslaw.
6. Serve and enjoy.

Ratatouille Spaghetti

Serves: 3

Ingredients:

- 1 Zucchini, chopped
- 1 Red Bell Pepper, chopped
- 1 Portobello Mushroom, chopped
- 1 Eggplant, sliced
- 1 cup Marinara Sauce
- 8 ounces Spaghetti
- 2 tsp chopped Basil
- 2 tbsp. Parmesan Cheese
- Salt, to taste

Method:

1. Sprinkle the eggplant slices with salt, and place them in a colander. Let sit for 15 minutes.
2. Preheat your grill to medium heat.
3. Grill the chopped veggies for about 10 minutes, or until tender.
4. Meanwhile, bring a pot with salted water to a boil over medium heat.
5. Add the spaghetti and cook according to the package's instructions.
6. Rinse and drain the pasta.
7. Toss the drained pasta and grilled veggies in a large bowl.
8. Divide between three serving bowls.
9. Top with chopped parsley and some parmesan cheese.
10. Enjoy.

Ground Beef Chile Relleno

Serves: 4

Ingredients:

- 8 ounces pureed Tomato
- 1 Red Onion, chopped
- 1 cup chopped Cilantro
- 1 tsp Olive Oil
- 1 1/2 tsp Chili Powder
- ½ pound ground Beef
- 6 ounces shredded Monterey Jack Cheese
- 2 Garlic Cloves, minced
- ½ tbsp. plus 1 tsp Cumin
- Salt and Pepper, to taste
- 4 Poblano Peppers

Method:

1. Brush the poblano peppers with olive oil, and place them under the broiler. Make sure to turn them around until their skin blackens.
2. Cover the peppers and let sit for 5 minutes.
3. When cooled slightly, peel them and discard the skins.
4. Add the beef and onion in a pan over medium heat, and cook until the beef is browned.
5. Add the garlic and cook for one more minute.
6. Stir in tomato puree, as well as the rest of the ingredients.
7. Stuff the poblano peppers with the beef mixture.
8. Place them in a baking pan.
9. Pour the tomato sauce over.
10. Bake at 350 degrees for about half an hour, or until bubbly.
11. Serve and enjoy.

Lentil and Potato Dahl

Serves: 4

Ingredients:

- 2 tbsp. Curry Powder
- 1 cup Red Lentils
- 3 Garlic Cloves, minced
- ½ Onion, diced
- 1 thumb-sized piece of Ginger, ground
- 1 Sweet Potato, diced
- 1 tbsp. Olive Oil
- 2 cups Water
- 1 Chili Pepper, deseeded and chopped
- 15 ounces canned Crushed Tomatoes
- Salt and Pepper, to taste

Method:

1. Heat the olive oil in a pot over medium heat.
2. Add the diced onions and potatoes and cook for 4 minutes.
3. Add pepper and ginger and cook for 2 more.
4. Add the garlic and cook for one more minute.
5. Stir in some salt and curry powder/
6. Stir in the lentils.
7. Add water, tomatoes, and season with some more salt.
8. Cover and let simmer for 20 minutes.
9. Serve and enjoy.

Beef Bourguignon

Serves: 6

Ingredients:

- 3 tbsp. Flour
- 1 pound Lean Beef, cut into chunks
- Two handfuls of Baby Shallots
- ½ pound Chestnut Mushrooms, halved
- 2 cups Red Wine
- 2 Bay Leaves
- 4 Carrots, peeled and sliced
- 1 tbsp. Olive Oil
- 2 Sprigs of Thyme
- 2 tbsp. chopped Parsley
- 1 2/3 cup Beef Broth

Method:

1. Preheat your oven to 320 degrees F.
2. Coat the beef with the flour.
3. Heat the olive oil in a casserole dish over medium heat.
4. Cook the beef until it is no longer pink on all sides.
5. Set aside.
6. Add carrots, onions, and mushrooms, and cook for 10 minutes.
7. Add the remaining ingredients and stir to combine well.
8. Cover the dish with a foil and place in the oven for 2 hours.
9. Serve and enjoy.

Pasta and Bean Skillet

Serves: 4

Ingredients:

- 1 cup Salsa
- 8 ounces Tomato Sauce
- ½ cup shredded Cheddar Cheese
- 2/3 cup Elbow Macaroni
- 2 tsp Chili Powder
- ¾ cup Water
- 2 cups Kidney Beans

Method:

1. Place all of the ingredients, except the cheese, in a non-stick skillet, and bring the mixture to a boil.
2. Cover the skillet and let simmer for 15 minutes or until the pasta is tender. Make sure to stir frequently.
3. Serve the pasta topped with shredded Cheddar cheese.
4. Enjoy.

3-Cheese Spinach Cannelloni

Serves: 6

Ingredients:

- 4 ½ ounces Mascarpone Cheese
- 24 ounces Frozen Spinach
- 12 ounces Pasta Sheets
- 12 ounces Ricotta Cheese
- 1 tsp Nutmeg
- 8 ounces Mozzarella Cheese plus 1 cup for topping
- A handful of Basil

Sauce

- ½ Onion, diced
- 28 ounces crushed Tomatoes
- 1 tsp Olive Oil A handful of Basil
- 4 Garlic Cloves, minced
- Salt, to taste

Method:

1. Heat the olive oil in a pan.
2. Add the onion and sauté for a couple of minutes.
3. Add garlic and sauté for another minute
4. Add tomatoes, basil, and season with some salt.
5. Preheat your oven to 350 degrees F.
6. Combine the spinach, cheeses some salt, and nutmeg.
7. Cut the pasta sheets in half.
8. Divide the filling between the pasta sheets and roll them up.
9. Pour half of the marinara sauce in the bottom of a baking dish.
10. Arrange the pasta rolls over.
11. Pour the remaining marinara sauce over, and top with mozzarella cheese.
12. Bake for about 45 minutes.
13. Serve and enjoy.

SNACKS

Orange Bowl Muesli

Serves: 6

Ingredients:

- 6 Empty Orange Halves, peel only (these will be the bowls)
- 2 cups Yogurt
- 1 ½ cups Rolled Oats
- 2 Apples, diced
- ½ cup sliced Almonds
- ½ tsp Cardamom
- Zest from 1 Lime
- ½ cup dried Cranberries
- 2 Clementine

Method:

1. Combine the oats, yogurt, zest, cardamom, apples, almonds, and dried cranberries in a bowl.
2. Fill the orange peel bowls with the mixture and refrigerate them overnight.
3. Serve topped with clementine slices and enjoy.

Tofu Lettuce Wraps

Serves: 4

Ingredients:

- 14 ounces cubed Tofu
- 1 tbsp. Rice Vinegar
- 1 tbsp. Tamari
- 2 tsp Coconut Oil
- 1 tbsp. Chili Sauce
- 2 tbsp. Sunflower Seeds
- 4 large Lettuce Leaves
- 1 Red Bell Pepper, cut into strips

Method:

1. Combine the tamari, chili sauce, and rice vinegar in a bowl.
2. Add the tofu, cover, and let marinate for 1 hour.
3. Melt the coconut oil in a skillet.
4. Add the tofu, and cook until browned about 5 minutes.
5. Divide the mixture between the lettuce leaves, top with red bell pepper slices and sunflower seeds, and roll them up.
6. Serve and enjoy.

Bacon and Blue Cheese Baked Cabbage

Serves: 4

Ingredients:

- 1 Head of Cabbage
- 3 ounces crumbled Blue Cheese
- 4 Slices of Bacon
- 1 tsp Olive Oil
- Salt, to taste
- Dressing:
- 1 Garlic Clove, minced
- 1 tsp Honey
- ¼ cup Olive Oil
- 1/2 minced Shallot
- 1 tsp Dijon Mustard
- Pinch of Salt

Method:

1. Preheat your grill to high heat.
2. Cut the cabbage in four. If your cabbage head is large, cut it into eights.
3. Brush the cabbage with some olive oil and sprinkle with salt.
4. Place the cabbage on the grill and grill for about 10 minutes on each side.
5. Meanwhile whisk all of the dressing ingredients together.
6. Place the bacon in a skillet over medium heat and cook it until crisp.
7. Crumble the cheese and bacon over the cabbage wedges.
8. Drizzle with the balsamic vinegar.
9. Serve and enjoy.

Almond Cranberry Energy Bites

Serves: 4

Ingredients:

- 1 cup Oatmeal
- 1 tbsp. Chia Seeds
- ¼ cup Honey
- ½ cup Peanut Butter
- 1/3 cup chopped Almonds
- 1 tbsp. Flaxseed
- 1/3 cup shredded Coconut, unsweetened
- 1/3 cup dried Cranberries

Method:

1. Preheat your oven to 350 degrees F.
2. Combine the oatmeal, coconut, and almonds, in a baking dish.
3. Place in the oven and cook for 10 minutes, stirring once halfway through.
4. Place the peanut butter in a microwave-safe bowl and microwave for about 20 seconds, until it becomes runny.
5. Place it in a bowl along with the rest of the ingredients.
6. Make 16 balls out of the mixture.
7. Serve and enjoy.

Black Bean Hummus

Serves: 6

Ingredients:

- 15 ounces canned Black Beans
- 1 tbsp. Olive Oil
- ½ cup Fresh Cilantro
- Juice of ½ Lemon
- 1 Garlic Clove, minced
- 1 tbsp. Tahini
- ½ Jalapeno
- A pinch of Salt

Method:

1. Place all of the ingredients in the bowl of your food processor.
2. Process for a minute or two, or until smooth.
3. Serve with veggies and crackers and enjoy.

Lemon Strawberry Shortcake Trifle

Serves: 1

Ingredients:

- 1 Lemon Bar, crumbled
- 1/3 cup low-fat Yogurt
- 1/3 cup Strawberries, sliced
- 1/3 cup sugar-free Instant Lemon Pudding

Method:

1. In a serving glass, add ½ of the yogurt, then add a layer of ½ of the pudding, and top with half of the strawberries and half of the lemon bar.
2. Repeat the layers one more time and enjoy a tasty and fruity snack.

Nacho Cupcakes

Serves: 12

Ingredients:

- 1 ½ cup Cornmeal
- ½ cup Sugar
- 1 cup chopped Chives
- 2 Eggs
- 1 cup of Buttermilk
- 1 ½ tsp Baking Powder
- ½ cup plus 2 tbsp. Flour
- ½ cup Milk
- ¼ cup chopped Jalapenos

Frosting

- ¼ cup Whipped Cream Cheese
- ¼ cup Crème Fraiche
- ¼ cup grated Monterey Jack Cheese
- Toppings:
- 12 Tortilla Chips
- 1 small Tomato, diced

Method:

1. Preheat your oven to 375 degrees F.
2. Combine all of the dry ingredients in one bowl, and whisk all of the wet ingredients in another.
3. Carefully combine the two mixtures, making sure that there aren't any lumps left.
4. Line your muffin tins and pour the batter into the pan. You can go ahead and fill them all the way to the top.
5. Place in the oven and bake for 20 minutes.
6. Meanwhile, combine the crème fraiche, Monterey Jack, and cream cheese, in a bowl.
7. Spread the topping over the cooked cupcakes.
8. Top the cupcakes with diced tomatoes and tortilla chips.

Cinnamon Rice Pudding

Serves: 6

Ingredients:

- 1 ¼ cup Water
- ¾ cup Basmati Rice
- 2 cups Milk
- ¼ tsp Nutmeg
- ½ cup Sugar
- A pinch of Salt
- 1 tsp Vanilla Extract
- 1 tbsp Butter
- 2 Cinnamon Sticks
- 1 Egg
- ½ tsp Cinnamon

Method:

1. Place the water in a pot over medium heat and bring to a boil.
2. Add rice and cook for about 15 minutes.
3. In another pot, add 1 ½ cups of milk, salt, sugar, and cinnamon sticks. Stir to combine well.
4. Place on low heat and cook until the sugar is completely dissolved.
5. Add the cooked rice into the mixture and cook for 20 minutes.
6. In a bowl, combine the remaining milk, cinnamon, egg, nutmeg, and vanilla extract.
7. Remove the pot from the heat and discard the cinnamon sticks.
8. Add some of the rice mixture into the bowl with cinnamon and vanilla milk.
9. Stir well, and then stir the entire bowl into the rice mixture.
10. Fold in the butter.
11. Pour the mixture into serving glasses, cover with plastic wrap, and refrigerate until set.
12. Serve and enjoy.

Energy Sandwich Bombs

Serves: 4

Ingredients:

- 4 Hawaiian Sweet Rolls
- 4 tbsp. Peanut Butter
- 2 tsp Honey
- 1 Banana, sliced

Method:

1. Cut the Hawaiian sweet rolls open.
2. Spread a tablespoon of peanut butter onto each roll.
3. Drizzle ½ tsp of honey over.
4. Top with slices of banana.
5. Close the roll and enjoy.

Conclusion

What are you waiting for? Clean your kitchen from the tempting junk food and other unhealthy ingredients and stack your fridge and shelves with the most nutritious superfoods for athletic performance.

Only by following the simple guidelines for balanced sports nutrition can you really reach your peak performance and grow as an athlete.

Preview of Triathlon Training by Matt Jordan

The Ultimate Guide for Boosting Performance, Improving Mental Toughness, and Gaining the Perfect Physical Condition for your Very First Triathlon

WHY SO DISCOURAGED?

And you thought running a marathon was intimidating. Triathlon, as the name suggests is a combination of three different sports. It is a discipline that is far trickier than signing up for a bike race, and it surely requires more training than preparing your body to endure the long mileage of a marathon. Triathlon is a competition that requires completion of three different and continuous disciplines: swimming, cycling and running back to back. And while you may think how signing for a triathlon can only throw discouragement your way, the truth is, when it comes to pushing your physical abilities and improving your athletic performance, there is no better way to do so. This competition is not that demanding so it can bring discouragement, but fulfillment.

Although it wasn't until the past few years that the Triathlon reached its well-known glory, the truth is, this competition is not that all new. The roots of Triathlon are set in the 1920s in France, where athletes used to participate in a race called "Les Trois Sports" meaning "The Three Sports". And as you've already guessed, yes, those three sports were swimming, cycling, and running. The participants had to swim across the Marne channel, then ride their bikes for 12 kilometers, and finish the race by taking a 3-kilometer run.

But it wasn't until the 70s rolled in when Triathlon was introduced to America. The very first Triathlon was held in San Diego on September 25, 1974, which is considered to be the official birthday of this demanding competition. And although at that time many disapproved this challenging event, the number of triathletes rapidly started growing after the Triathlon debut at the Sydney Olympic Games in 2000.

Now, I don't know if you want to become an Olympian or you simply want to push your physical endurance a little bit farther, but I know becoming a triathlete doesn't have to be so downright discouraging. There is nothing that cannot be achieved with the right amount of preparation, motivation, and training, and luckily for you, these next chapters hold the secret about how to cross the Triathlon's finish line.

If you enjoyed this preview, please visit:
https://www.amazon.com/dp/B073YHRMPR/

Printed in Great Britain
by Amazon